TREASURES

OF THE

HEART

TREASURES
OF THE
HEART

Theckedath Mathew, M.D.

VANTAGE PRESS
New York

The opinions and instructions expressed herein are solely those of the author. Each individual should seek the advice of his or her own physician before starting any new medical program.

To my loving wife Susan,
my children Nisha, Sheena, and Ajay.
Thank you for your unconditional
love and support.

Acknowledgment

I dutifully acknowledge the beautiful work done by Lori Hasman in preparation of this manuscript and my daughter Sheena Mathew for her editorial assistance.

Dedication

I am thankful to the many thousands of patients whom I had the great privilege to be acquainted with, consulted on, and provided treatment for along with many other procedures. Representing all my patients I submit this book to Carmine Ciccarone, a survivor of sudden cardiac arrest. (Carmine's story is on page 101).

I would like to record my special thanks to a few of my teachers who guided and crafted my career. Shree I.D. Chacko, B.A.L.T., of St. Mary's High School, Kuravilangad; Professor Joy Joseph of St. Berchman's College; Professor P.J. Geevarghese, Professor K.J. Jacob, Professor George Jacob, and Professor Mary Phillips from my medical school; Professor Rudolph Napodano, my program director from the University of Rochester; Professor Navin Nanda for all the echocardiography I know; and Dr. J. Hollaman of Cleveland Clinic, Ohio, for giving me the opening lessons in angioplasty.

"Knowledge is experience
Everything else is just information"

Albert Einstein

Edited by

Selvakumar Chockalingam, M.D.

Contents

Contents

Foreword

It is a great pleasure and privilege for me to write about Dr. Theckedath Mathew and his book *Treasures of the Heart*. My association with Theckedath goes back to over twenty years ago when he came to work with me to learn the then developing technique of echocardiography (cardiac ultrasound). Even at that time I was impressed with his hard work and scholarship, but moreso with the caring attitude that he displayed toward his patients. Our relationship at that time was more as friends rather than as teacher-student and I have cherished that relationship ever since.

Dr. Mathew has practiced medicine on four different continents: Asia, Africa, Europe, and the Americas, and the book details his personal experiences in dealing with patients in many countries, including the U.S.A. The book is very well written and I became so absorbed in reading it that I could not bring myself to put it down until I had finished reading the last page. The book also demonstrates not only Dr. Mathew's expertise in cardiology, but also his kindness, compassion, and humanitarian attitude toward his patients.

This book is a storehouse of knowledge for the general public and patients, especially those with cardiac problems, and I recommend it be placed in every physician's waiting room library.

—Navin C. Nanda, M.D.
Professor of Medicine and
Director, Heart Station/Echocardiography Laboratories
The University of Alabama at Birmingham

Preface

I had the great privilege and opportunity to learn, practice, and teach the art and science of medicine in four continents of the world, Asia, Africa, Europe, and the United States of America. While the common denominator in each of these continents is to heal the sick, the approach, reasoning, resources, philosophy, and the principles of medical practice are astonishingly different in class and kind.

Based on my personal observations and hands-on experience, I am convinced that the medical practice in the United States holds the highest standards of all; though painfully plagued by frivolous lawsuits and exorbitant waste in attempting to provide high-tech medicine particularly for end-stage medical conditions. The story of the 40 million or so Americans without any medical insurance is un-American to say the least. Let me give you a glimpse of my experience in medical practice abroad, just to compare and contrast it with our own system.

The year was 1966.

I was a 3rd year medical student at Kottayam Medical College in Kerala, India, doing Internal Medicine clinical clerkship. A 12-year-old girl named Mary was brought to me with the complaints of fever, heavy sweats, vomiting, diarrhea, and weight loss over two weeks. This girl with a pale angelic face looked frail and dehydrated, had sunken eyes, clammy skin, a fast thready pulse, and shallow breathing with frequent episodes of apnea. My close friend John Valliatu and I tried to locate a venous access for the administration of fluids but failed. Then, we performed a brachial venous cut down, and administered a large amount of Ringer lactate solution. She had advanced typhoid fever. I knew Mary's family from before. Her father was a lower-middle-class farmer from a remote village without electricity or telephones. He worked in the paddy fields, and grew a thick lush of coconut trees, arrack nut trees, black peppers, and coffee around his small tiled house that had a well for drinking water in the front courtyard.

In Kerala, the thunderous downpour of a monsoon had just settled down. As usual, there was the annual mini-epidemic of cholera and other infectious diseases. The limited hospital beds were full and overflowing. In the general medical wards, between two regular beds, we created a "floor bed" for Mary by placing a mattress on the floor with a pillow and bare minimum sheets. She was treated with intravenous fluids, chloramphenicol, and other supportive medications. The family went back home leaving her overall care under my responsibility.

The next day Mary felt better. She spoke a few words, smiled, asked for her younger sister, and even drank some rice soup. Around midnight I received a call from the head nurse of the medical floor who informed me that the child was found dead in her sleep. With my friend John we went to the medical floor. The nurses had put a nice dress on her, combed her hair, cleaned her body, and prepared her to be transferred. I had no way to contact the family, and the only two ambulances in town that carried dead bodies were unavailable that night. I did not want to leave the little girl with the angelic face encased in the hospital morgue with the horrible pungent smell of formalin and decaying bodies. It was not the right place for Mary, although that would not have bothered her at all.

My friend John came to me with a plan. "Mathacha," he said.

"We will take Mary in a taxicab and pretend that she is sleeping." I readily agreed to this plan. Within minutes, we were in the rear seat of a taxicab, with Mary on our laps, embarking on an 18-mile trip through the country roads, which took over one hour. We had a plan to present Mary to her family. About a half a mile before Mary's home, around 3:00 a.m. in the morning, I went to the home of a man I knew well, woke him up, and told him the whole story. He agreed to go to Mary's house in advance with two of his neighbors to deliver the tragic news, and prepare Mary's family to receive her body. The country road ended about 500 yards short of Mary's home. John walked in front of me with a flashlight through the muddy banks of a little creek, and I followed him with Mary on my shoulders. The family with a few neighbors in heavy sobbing received Mary from my hands. Mary's mother and two siblings cried out loud, and her father stood there motionless. John and I went back to the hospital in the same taxicab.

After my graduate training in medical school, I went to Africa for a teaching assignment, and then moved to the United Kingdom, and finally to the United States for higher studies. However, I visited my home every year. On most of those occasions, Mary's father was there at the airport to receive me, and to thank me again and again with his usual presents of fruits, nuts, honey, and other country goods.

The year was 1972.

I was working as a Registrar in medicine at the University Teaching Hospital in Lusaka, Zambia. I was preparing for the board exam of the Royal College of Physicians in London. One of the prerequisites to sit for the exam was to have a minimum of six months' of training at the Senior House Officer Level in either surgery or obstetrics/gynecology. I opted to work in the OB/GYN unit.

The University Teaching Hospital at Lusaka is one of the largest hospital complexes in the world; it was built at a time when the price of copper was sky high. In its hey-days, up to 1800 physicians worked in the hospital around-the-clock. The OB/GYN unit served a geographic area of over a 100-mile radius. We had 22 delivery rooms and 6 OR suites. The whole atmosphere was filled with the rhythmic cacophonous music of delivering mothers' oohs and cries, the nurses' "push...push," and the newborn babies screams and squeals.

Within the first few hours of my assignment to the unit, I delivered babies, performed episiotomies, and even forceps deliveries. The remainder of the day I assisted on three or four cesarean sections. My unit chief and supervisor was an extremely arrogant South African Asian. However, he noticed that I was "a very skilled surgeon." He profusely complimented the way I took the suture bites and tied the knots. His wife was a senior Registrar in the unit, and had the responsibility to stay in the hospital while she was on-call. However, because I was so very "capable," my supervisor decided that I could handle any situations in the hospital with the rest of the House Staff, and that his wife would not have to stay in the hospital at night any more. He assured me that they would be available by phone should any problems arise that I could not handle. I was thrilled at my instant fame, apparent "seniority," and the professor's public citation of my skills.

About three weeks later I saw a 40-year-old mother weighing over 300 pounds, who claimed that she was over 11 months pregnant.

She was in pain and could not lie down flat. Her tummy billowed down to one side, and the umbilicus was at the level of her knees. She appeared toxic, and there was clearly evidence of fetal distress. Around 7:00 p.m., the decision was made to perform an emergency cesarean section. Despite my pleadings and apparent inexperience to handle such a case, my supervisor assured me that things would be just fine, and he instructed me to, "proceed step-by-step as I have taught you." The surgery started. I made a large incision on the abdomen, dissected through the adipose, and eventually found the abdominal rectus fascia about half a foot in depth. Then, I separated the rectus muscle, dissected the peritoneum and reached the abdominal cavity, and delivered the baby via an incision of the uterus. The baby was alive, and we in the OR all sighed with relief for a moment…but only for a moment. The deep abdominal cavity was soon filled with blood. I searched for the source of bleeding. It was not from the incision site, but from somewhere very deep in the pelvic cavity. I tried to pack the lower abdomen with numerous thick gauzes only to see that fresh blood was gushing at me with a vengeance. I sent an S.O.S. to my supervisor, but there was no return call. The patient's blood pressure was bottoming-out. We gave her several units of blood. With my four weeks of OB/GYN surgical experience, I was virtually helpless, nervous, and was sweating. In situations like this I usually pray to all the gods I know to send me a guardian angel. In my mind I conjured up the image of a Byzantine iconographic painting of St. Mary with baby Jesus in her lap, a 15th Century painting that hung on the altar of my village church, which was so engraved in my mind "or soul" from my early childhood days as an altar boy. Moments felt like hours. God forbid! Then there appeared a guardian angel at the door, Professor Gulshan, another OB/GYN Unit Chief in the same department. "What seems to be the problem boy", he called out. Holding a surgical mask over his face he came near the OR table, tiptoeing, and looked at the scene. In a resoundingly loud, confident and thick voice he ordered, "Put your hand behind the fundus of the uterus and lift it up." I did exactly what he said, and then everything became so clear and visible to me. I saw the tear on the lower end of the uterus extending to the left broad ligament that severed the uterine artery causing blood to profusely spurt to 10-inches in height. I felt so very happy when I saw that bloody spurter. With great joy and relief I caught that spot with an artery forceps. The bleeding stopped. The rest of the case was a piece of cake.

The next morning my supervisor made rounds in the hospital. He made no apologies for not coming to help me or seeing the patient that night. He told me that I did an outstanding job...I really hated that man, so much so that I never showed up for a farewell dinner he arranged for me when I left the unit.

The year was 1974.

I was working as a Medical Registrar at the Preston Hall Regional Cardiothoracic Center in Maidstone, United Kingdom. My friend Dr. V. John (the British called him Mister John, as he was a Fellow of the Royal College of Surgeons of London by that time) was working in the same CT unit. I enjoyed the way the British practiced medicine. They knew the limitations of their resources, and utilized them in a highly appropriate way.

Around the beginning of December 1974, I admitted a 74-year-old veteran with his second heart attack, congestive heart failure, and recurrent ventricular tachycardia. He had traveled extensively in Europe, India, China, Africa, and the Americas. He had a hacking productive cough of chronic bronchitis, like a good many of the

British have. He used to narrate all kinds of stories in an engrossing way whenever he had a chance in between the defibrillations and resuscitations. After a couple of days, he decided not to have any more procedures. He spoke little of his family, a will, or anything of that nature. He was so content with life. On each and every occasion he thanked us for anything and everything we did. It appeared to me that he even knew the exact time of his death. He told me that his stay at Preston Hall was only for a day or two, but certainly not more than three. The next day in my evening rounds I sat by his side and held his arms and chatted for a while. He was sipping a lager (which was a norm in British hospitals). In a thick, but soft, voice he told me that his son, the only living relative, was a big businessman in London. "When I am gone," he emphasized, "then only does my son need to be informed of my stay here at Preston Hall. Please tell him that I was a good patient," he insisted. He talked about his tour of duty in India, his hunting adventures, and experiences with fortunetellers, army rum, spicy foods and the sepoy girls. He also told me that he would save a trip for Santa that year, as he was planning to meet him up at the North Pole pretty soon. Pretty soon it was, as he was pronounced dead the next day. Sure enough I told his son that his father indeed was a great patient.

It was Rochester, New York, in the mid 1980s.

I got a call from the ER physician of a small community hospital about a 72-year-old, longstanding hypertensive and diabetic man, with a history of heavy cigarette smoking, who was being admitted with severe unstable angina. I saw the patient immediately. He had acute coronary syndrome with mild congestive cardiac failure. His EKGs were suggestive of a nontransmural myocardial infarction, and his cardiac pumping function had dropped from a normal of 65%

to 30%. He was treated quite appropriately with oxygen, aspirin, intravenous Nitroglycerin, Heparin, beta blockers, Digoxin, and diuretics. He had recurrent episodes of chest pain during the night, and had received several doses of Morphine.

The next morning I saw the patient and made some fine-tuning in his medications, and called for a family conference. The ICU head nurse, Ms. Peggy Hurst, was an experienced and highly respected person. She advised me to be especially careful with the family, and that the patient's wife was already talking about possible lawsuits. Extremely careful that I was, I held a detailed conference with the patient's family in the presence of the ICU head nurse. I told the family that the patient had severe unstable angina with evidence of myocardial infarction and heart failure. Since he had already been given the maximum medical management at this stage, the next step would be to consider transferring him to Rochester General Hospital to explore the options of intra-aortic balloon pump, coronary angiography, and the possibility of coronary artery bypass graft surgery. I explained the risks and benefits of the procedures at length with the help of diagrams and pictures. Approximately an hour later, a second conference was held with the patient and his family, in the presence of the ICU head nurse. Thereafter, I was advised by the family to proceed with the plans for a coronary angiogram.

He was taken to the tertiary care hospital. The coronary angiography held no surprises. He had very severe three-vessel coronary artery disease with an ejection fraction of 30%, with continued chest pain. An intra-aortic balloon pump was inserted. The cardiac surgeons examined the patient, reviewed the angiogram, and another family conference was held. All were in agreement to proceed to an emergency CABG. While the patient was being trollied to the OR, he developed a massive stroke and died.

The Chief of Medicine, with whatever little cardiology he knew, reviewed the case, and cited me for performing an unnecessary high-risk procedure that created considerable liability for the hospital. I explained to him that what I did was absolutely right, and that if I had to do it again I would do it exactly the same. I also stated that tertiary care hospitals are meant to and have the duty to handle such high-risk patients if deemed necessary. I knew my decisions were clinically sound and ethically right. However, the "Chief," a soft-spoken and ambitious hypocrite, told the "Indian" (in many different words) that he hated my guts, and that he was willing to endanger my licensure to practice medicine, all because I wanted to do the very best for that man. Unwilling to prostrate myself in front of his feet, I told the Chief that he must do whatever he thought was right.

It was the single most unpleasant event in my whole professional career. I had several sleepless nights and sexless weeks. My wife and family were extremely upset. I got into two minor car accidents that same month. Finally, I took a trip downtown and saw a couple of senior attorneys. They were simply dismayed at the "Chief's" attitude and comments. They assured me, "Doctor, for this case, if anything happens to your license…you can have a comfortable and early retirement." I went on with my business of practicing good medicine as I always did.

God forbid, within eight weeks after the incident there was a letter from the patient's attorney charging me with negligence, carelessness, performing procedures without informed consent from either the patient or family, transferring the patient to another hospital without permission, administering wrong medications, and performing balloon procedures not within the standards of care, which together culminated in the death of the patient. Then, the day of my deposition arrived. It was quite an enjoyable treat for me. The plaintiff's attorney questioned me for eight and a half hours. At times he appeared somewhat rude and intimidating for which I had no problem with, as I knew my trade a touch better than he knew his own. My attorney was really thrilled at my precise, apt, and, at times, stingingly sarcastic answers.

Soon after, the medical liability insurance company requested that I settle this case out of court for a "small amount of money." It was financially beneficial for them to settle rather than pay the attorney's fees, even if it resulted in a black mark on my records. I believed in my convictions and hoped that true justice would not defy me. In fact, I told the insurance company that I would settle if the plaintiff was willing to compensate me for my pain and suffering. Finally, the case was unconditionally dismissed against me, and the case was closed.

The above case is a somewhat isolated incident, and is not at all a reflection of the overall practice of medicine in the United States. However, I am convinced that there are quite a large number of frivolous lawsuits creating an aura of paranoia in the medical profession. This has resulted in a culture of practicing "defensive medicine" at the cost of conducting a large number of unnecessary tests and procedures. Medicine is an art based on the scientific facts, and a lot of common sense and ethics.

Based on my three decades of experience spread over four continents, I can say that we here in the United States practice the principles of medicine the best in the world, but the cost is enormous. The considerable waste of ordering numerous tests and unnecessary procedures saddens me. There must be a reasonable limit in the utilization of our resources. On one end of the spectrum, we have children who are not immunized, and 40 million Americans without any medical insurance coverage. On the other end of the spectrum, we spend about 100 billion dollars for the last three months of the patient's life. At times, it appears to me that the medical community is always trying "at any cost" to prolong the inevitable truth of death, especially when a segment of the patient community wants to believe that disease and death are consequences of some wrongdoing by somebody. As it turns out, in many instances, all these tests and procedures are good enough only to establish a clinical diagnosis or clarify a medical cause of death without a postmortem examination, at the cost of prolongation of the terminal state by a few days or weeks at the very best. But we as patients and caregivers must be reminded at times that death is the result of birth itself. There is something called "natural causes" of death, which cannot be circumvented by any amount of stenting, CABG, or organ transplantations. We, as a community, have to learn to focus and target our resources for the needed cause. We have to groom a health-conscious community. We must focus a lot more on the preventive aspects of diseases, in addition to early detection and timely interventions.

Many times when I talk to my patients about commonplace issues in cardiovascular diseases it occurs to me that some of these facts and instructions strike them as a surprise, as it does to many health care workers and even some physicians. In this small book I touch base with a variety of clinical situations, epidemiology, treatment modalities, and above all individual and community responsibilities pertaining to cardiovascular problems. The four cases briefly mentioned above are excerpts from my book in preparation for *The Odyssey of an Ordinary Man.*

The Book

*I love the concept of **"the book"** as it is so objective, handy, academic, transportable even through an airport security system, and you may indulge into at any given moment of your choice with no hard- or software required; you can hold it all the time, breathe into it, and finally make a friend out of it. And above all, I can converse with you one-on-one with no commercial interruptions.*

The Author

Introduction

In its abruptness, unpredictability, and savage toll on human life, acute myocardial infarction is second to none in terms of the afflictions known to mankind.

Cardiovascular disease continues to be the leading and most menacing medical problem in the United States. Fifty-eight million Americans, i.e., approximately one in every five Americans, are affected by coronary artery disease (CAD), hypertension or stroke, all collectively called cardiovascular diseases (CVD). Acute myocardial infarction (AMI), also known as heart attack or heart seizure, strikes 1.5 million Americans annually. In spite of the phenomenal developments in medical science at prohibitive costs, we still lose about 500,000 lives to coronary heart disease every year. Unfortunately, about 250,000 amongst this group die before reaching a hospital.

In the United States, since the National Heart, Lung, and Blood Institute was established in 1948, and started tracking the incidence of coronary artery disease; it had reached epidemic proportions in the 1950s. The incidence of CAD peaked in the 1960s, and is now on the decline.

In fact, the death rate from CAD has dropped by 68% from 1960 to 1998. The decline has been quite dramatic in the last ten years. From 1995 to 1998, coronary deaths have declined by 3.6% each year. The incidence of transmural myocardial infarcts has declined, although the incidence of nontransmural myocardial infarction has increased.

This decline is mostly from advanced and aggressive in-hospital care of patients and post-discharge management. In-hospital mortality has gone down from 36% in 1980 to approximately 9% now.

At present, we are proud to say that our medical system provides the very best care to AMI patients on the planet. The introduction of highly effective clot-buster medications ($1300-$2500 per dose), emergency angioplasty ($14,000-$18,000 per patient), and similar interventions has really revolutionized the treatment of AMI. In the 1960s and early 1970s, a patient with an acute myocardial infarction when admitted to the hospital was prescribed bed rest for a minimum of two weeks, along with a liquid diet, painkillers and other sedatives. An electrocardiogram was recorded once a day for the first couple of days, and thereafter once every few days. Virtually none of the patients were considered for coronary angiography or other revascularization procedures.

Over the past 30 years, the management of acute myocardial infarction has been revolutionized with the introduction of sophisticated pharmacological and other technological devices, such as powerful rhythm-controlling medications, beta blockers, aspirin, angiotensin converting enzyme inhibitors, automated defibrillators, etc. In the early 1980s, another powerful tool, popularly known as clot-blusters, came into use. We started treating patients with acute myocardial infarction in the earliest possible minutes with these powerful clot-blusters, reestablishing the blood flow in a clogged blood vessel, and ultimately saving several thousand lives per year. However, the use of clot-busters is limited to a selected minority of patients. (See the insert: The myth of clot-busters, on page 29.) Subsequently, early angiography, coronary angioplasty, and stenting came into effect. With the advent of these treatment modalities, the patient fared immensely better when compared to previous treatment procedures. The in-hospital mortality of patients with acute myocardial infarction dropped from a staggering 33% to about 9%. Today, it is not unusual that if an acute myocardial infarction patient reaches the hospital **early enough**, he/she receives a clot-buster treatment or emergency angioplasty leading to rapid stabilization, early mobilization, and returning home as a productive member of the community by the third or fourth day. Yet, this phenomenal improvement in the quality of care has resulted in an overwhelming increase in healthcare expenditures. The overall economic impact of CVD treatment is a staggering $160 billion per year in the United States.

We can pretty much say that this has been the Golden Age of medicine in the United States, where the patient has had the privilege to see a physician or a specialist of his/her choice, and receive state-of-the-art medicine, though at high costs. However, the legacy of this great American medical practice will soon be history.

Today business ethics revolve around the allure of quarterly earnings rather than the laws of morality or the wisdom of collectivism. This type of quarterly earning-oriented business employers and profit-oriented medical business organizations have joined hands, and have concocted a health care rationing authority, otherwise known as the Health Maintenance Organizations (HMOs) to do the job of slaughtering our treasured social agenda of private practice in medicine. The greed and ruthlessness that hallowed the Wall Street for the last two decades is palpably evident amongst our for-profit HMOs. The long and short of the story is that medical care will be trimmed, slimmed, rationed, and dehydrated to make it simply cheap. Such cost-cutting measures are no more explicit than in the cardinal field of cardiovascular disease. In this strange environment, it is mandatory that we focus our attention to individuals, family, and community-at-large for the prevention and timely intervention in CVD affecting our community.

post on her wall at www.facebook.com/Susan.Aylworth.Author. "If you enjoy my books, please tell everyone you know: friends, relatives, neighbors, the person who delivers your mail, people you meet in line in the grocery store, everyone!" She welcomes ideas for new books and characters.

Eastward to Zion is eligible for a Whitney Award during the year of its publication. If you find it deserving, you may nominate it, or other books by LDS authors, at http://whitneyawards.com/wordpress/nominate. Thank you for reading.

Chapter One

Case Studies

 herewith denote the case histories of three of our community members who sustained acute cardiac events, received commensurable levels of primary as well as tertiary care, yet resulted in antipodal outcome.

Case I

It was about 6:00 p.m. when I received a call on my cell phone while driving back home from the day's work. The caller was my friend's wife, a staff nurse, and she was at work in one of the nearby hospitals.

"Dr. Mathew." She was sobbing and at times choking, but the words were clear and loud. "My husband is down on the floor in the kitchen. The paramedics are already there...They have been working on him for the past few minutes...Please come."

"O.K., I am on my way. I will meet you at the emergency room." There I started not knowing exactly where to go...to the emergency room or directly to their home. The man who was on the floor is a friend of mine. Barely five days back he was at my home to discuss a program for an upcoming social event. His wife was under my care for mild hypertension. I never knew that my friend had any medical problems at all, although a bit later I learned that he too had moderate hypertension and that his primary care physician was treating him with Procardia as monotherapy.

This S.O.S. call from the staff nurse came as a shock and was difficult to comprehend. Why didn't the paramedics take him to the emergency room; "Is he already dead? Yet, they have to take him to the ER, why this delay." I called the ER. He had not arrived there. I drove straight to their home with the blinkers on.

There he was on the floor blue and flaccid haloed by the paramedics in full cardiopulmonary resuscitation. The paramedics had established an intravenous line and he was intubated with assisted-breathing by an Ambu bag. However, he had no pulse or blood pressure. The EKG showed occasional escape beats and external cardiac massage was in progress for at least ten minutes. I participated in the CPR, gave additional medications, and defibrillated him a few more times. Thank God he responded with a decent pulse and blood pressure. The EKG showed evidence of a large anterior myocardial infarction. The patient clenched on the endotracheal tube and he certainly had a gag reflex. I alerted the cardiac catheterization call team, and planned for an emergency coronary angiography and possible intervention.

The ambulance was on the way to the hospital. I learned that he had some epigastric discomfort since approximately 10:00 a.m. that day. He self medicated with antacids initially and aspirin subsequently. He didn't eat lunch and was somewhat restless. He never had chest pain or shortness of breath. His 13-year-old son was at home and they conversed on several subjects in the territory of quality family time. By about 5:30 p.m. the epigastric burning intensified, he broke out into a massive sweat. At that particular moment he experienced intense chest pressure, became dizzy, foggy, and collapsed onto the floor. The upset and frightened son made the 911-call. The dialogue with the dispatch operator was somewhat protracted, and the ambulance reached the front door of their house in about 13 minutes. Some 7-8 minutes late for the community's standards. Those few minutes the sobbing, helpless boy spent with his loving father on the floor, breathless and motionless, is just inexplicable, and I can only hope that no child or family member ever has to endure such scenes. But the fact that similar scenes of climax are in the drama of human life are enacted and re-enacted only too frequently in our abodes and all across the world.

The ambulance reached the hospital in 15 minutes. The immensely talented Cath Lab Team had the room all prepared and ready to go. As expected, the cardiac catheterization revealed a single ruptured plaque located in the mid portion of the left anterior descending coronary artery (Fig. 1A). Most likely this artery was totally occluded at the beginning of the major event, some 60 minutes back. Now the body's own clot-lysing system with the help of the medications administered had recanalized the artery leaving some 90% residual stenosis. The insult to the left ventricle—the main pumping chamber of the heart—was minimal. The clogged artery was now opened by an angioplasty balloon catheter and then stented with a metallic slotted tube establishing excellent antegrade flow (Fig. 1B). His heart rate and blood pressure were quite stable thereafter, and he was transferred to the Coronary Care Unit.

I held a family conference with the immediate family and reviewed the clinical scenario, and cautioned that the final outcome entirely depends on the return of cerebral function. The family and friends stayed around his bed most of the night hoping that he would open his eyes and show some signs of hope. My friend did not wake up the next day or the five days thereafter.

The beacon of hope flickered and faded off. By the sixth day brain death was established beyond doubt. With the consensus of the family, physicians, and a priest of their congregation, artificial life support measures were discontinued and he was pronounced dead.

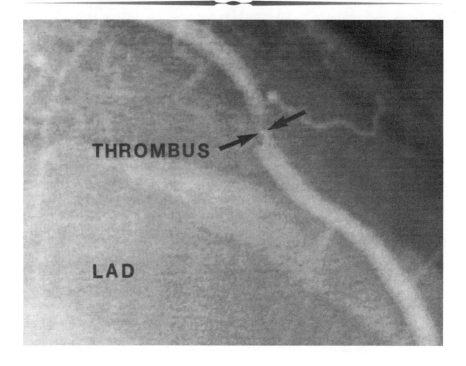

(**Fig. 1A**)   Selective left coronary angiography showing a blockage in the left anterior descending artery (LAD).

This lesion is a ruptured plaque with thrombus. Most likely
this artery was totally occluded at the beginning of the heart attack.
Now about 80 minutes later, the patient's own clot-lysing mechanism,
and the medications have recanalized the blockage. However, there is
a 90% blockage which limits blood flow, with a high likelihood of
reocclusion.

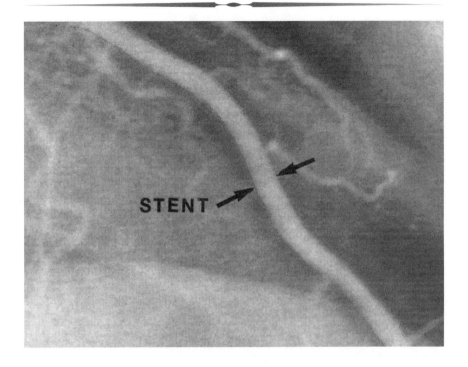

(**Fig. 1B**) The LAD after stenting. The lesion is now tacked up. Excellent antegrade flow is established.

The clogged artery was opened by a balloon angioplasty catheter and was stented (with a metallic coil) establishing excellent antegrade flow. His heart rate and blood pressure were quite stable thereafter.

Case II

A 48-year-old obese man with sedentary habits, who was also a heavy smoker with a family history of coronary heart disease, did not "feel well" on a Saturday afternoon. Following a light dinner, he felt nauseous. Due to the insistence of his wife, he agreed to go to the emergency room. Upon arrival to the hospital, he had moderate shortness of breath and chest pain. An acute evolving myocardial infarction was diagnosed,

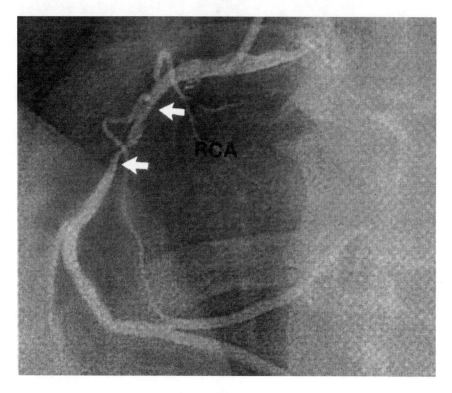

(**Fig. 2A**) Selective right coronary angiography of patient in Case II. The proximal and mid portions of the RCA are ulcerated with 70-90% stenosis.
RCA—right coronary artery.

and he received several medications including a clot-buster. His chest pain resolved, and his general condition was stable the first night. However, the next morning the chest pain recurred. He was then transferred to a tertiary care center, where he had an angiogram and angioplasty.

His cardiac condition stabilized quite well, enough to be discharged the next day. The patient received quite elaborate instructions and explanations pertaining to diet, exercise,

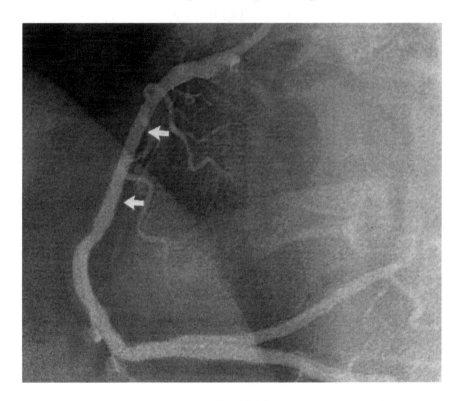

(**Fig. 2B**) RCA stenting. The blockage is now treated with deployment of a coronary stent. The RCA lumen now appears open, smooth, and normal.

smoking cessation, medications, and follow-up care, and returned to the community as a productive member.

The patients in Case I and Case II share a lot in common in terms of the etiology, symptoms, and pathology of their ailments. Both of them had acute myocardial infarctions; however, they both had atypical presentations without any crushing chest pain. The patient in Case I had rapid deterioration of his condition and lost a few valuable moments, approximately 13 minutes, before effective help reached his home. His initial presentation of AMI with epigastric discomfort was highly misleading, and therefore help was not sought earlier on, resulting in his loss of life.

Case III

It was spring in full bloom in upstate New York. The patient in focus was a healthy 54-year-old female with no cardiac risk factors, but did smoke four to five cigarettes per day. She had no significant past medical or surgical history, except for a flulike syndrome approximately four months back. The recollection of the case, as narrated by the patient's husband, reads as follows:

"This incredible experience, the profound images, sensations, and memories represent the most significant emotional event of my life."

Sunday, May 2, 1999

The weather was beautiful during the weekend; a great spring, unseasonably warm, as was the whole month of May. Saturday was very normal, Eileen went for her walk, and I ran 21 miles with Bill and Joel Allen in preparation for the Burlington Marathon. We had a barbecue in the backyard, and enjoyed the outdoors. The yard and the gardens were off to a great start.

On Sunday we were so excited about the weather we decided to go to Sara's Farm Market in Brockport to buy our annual plants. We planted pink and red wax begonias with white alyssum around the trees in the east lawn. Eileen did not complain about feeling ill, nor did she appear to be sick. We went to bed at our normal time around 9:00 p.m. to read, and fell asleep shortly thereafter.

Monday, May 3, 1999

4:00 a.m. At about this time I awoke to Eileen's light cough, not unusual because she was a light smoker; then, I heard one muffled guttural sound like she was choking. I nudged her, but she did not respond. Then, I reached over her, and turned on the lamp, and saw her frozen face. Her jaw was locked, mouth and eyes were closed, and she was flaccid and powerless as I tried to lift her arms. As I screamed at her, "Eileen, wake up" and to our daughter "Megan, call 911," my first thought was that she was choking on her tongue, so I tried to clear her tongue from her airway. After checking her airway, and getting bit by her clenched jaw, I rolled her to her side and tried the Heimlich maneuver to force out whatever may be in her throat. Nothing came out. Her body was limp and unresponsive despite my attempts to wake her. I began mouth-to-mouth resuscitation with one powerful breath of air. Although never formally trained, I had to try something. Eileen's chest responded to the air slightly, which was the only movement she ever made during this episode.

4:08 a.m.   Megan, after running to our bedroom door and screaming, "Daddy, what's wrong with mommy," very responsibly went to the boys' room and dialed 911. She informed the 911 operator that Eileen was not breathing and not responding.

4:09 a.m.   Upon her return to the hallway, I asked Megan to run across the street to our neighbor's house to get Eric Bradshaw, who is trained in CPR. In the meantime, Tommy O'Hearn, a village policeman, heard the 911 call, and raced to our house. For some reason Eric's wife Karen heard Megan's footsteps on their porch and woke Eric immediately. Eric and Megan were coming back across the street as Tommy arrived at our house.

4:10 a.m.   Although not counting or checking Eileen's pulse, I continued to breathe into her. When Eric and Tommy arrived I told them that my breaths were the only thing she had responded to and asked them to perform CPR.

4:12 a.m.   Tommy radioed to the dispatcher that CPR was in progress and that he felt a slight pulse (~40). Megan called our son Brian in Holley and asked him to come quickly.

4:13 a.m.   The Central Orleans Volunteer Ambulance crew (Ken Nunnery, Jena Korz, and Jeff Eisenheimer), were there at my door at 4:13 a.m. In addition, Nick Condolucci, the COVA Director of Operations, was on his way to work, and Keith Hale, a full-time paramedic in Rochester, who was also on his way to work, heard the call and arrived at our house by 4:15 a.m. Peter Sidari, an Albion fireman and my children's religious education instructor, arrived and supported Megan and myself in prayer.

4:15 a.m.   The ambulance crew took over CPR and started supporting Eileen's breathing with a mask and bag, and moved Eileen to the floor. They pushed the furniture back to make room for the crew and equipment. They checked her vitals and connected her to the monitor. Eileen was in cardiac arrest, the monitor showing that her heart was in ventricular fibrillation. They delivered a first shock, which she did not respond to. So Keith Hale checked her airway with a scope, checked her pupils, and then administered an IV drug. By this time Eileen's stomach was distended, her color was not good, and the situation was very scary.

The only thing that I could do was to pray and keep telling Eileen, "Come on baby, you can do it" repeatedly. Brian and Casey arrived within a few minutes, and the children tried to contact Don, our son, at college.

4:18 a.m.   They shocked Eileen again, and she responded with a heart rate of 120 beats per minute. The crew stabilized her, moved her to a backboard, and I helped them carry her down the stairs to the waiting ambulance.

4:40 a.m.   The ambulance left for Lakeside Hospital in Brockport, and I got dressed to follow the ambulance with Megan, Brian, and Casey.

5:00 a.m. At Lakeside Hospital Emergency Room, they already moved Eileen into the first bay before I could see her, and I was directed to admissions. The emergency room crew including Dr. Ellie, nurse Darcy Luzak, and P.A. Tom Stansiwicki stabilized Eileen and placed her on a respirator, and the ambulance crew remained on standby for a transfer if required. We all hung on as family members arrived, and we shared our emotions and prayers.

In a short time, the ambulance crew began packing up to leave. The bay curtain had not been opened, and I recall the fear of not knowing Eileen's condition. Then, she was wheeled out into the hallway, and I was asked to follow them for x-rays and a CAT scan on the way to the ICU. Eileen was turned over to Pat Moran, the ICU nurse, and a respiratory technician in the ICU. Eileen was fighting the respirator, so the decision was made to sedate her.

7:20 a.m. Dr. Charles Gelia briefed me on the initial diagnosis. Eileen's white blood cell count was over 20,000 (normal is 6,000 to 11,000), which indicated that there was an infection that probably involved the heart and lungs. Her heart was abnormal in size. The infection was probably as a result of a virus. Dr. Gelia had quickly assembled an expert team including Dr. Theckedath Mathew, cardiologist; Dr. Christian Brondon, pulmonologist; Dr. Al Dehar, Infection Disease specialist; Dr. David Marzulo, neurologist; and Dr. Kasaraneni, Director of Emergency Medicine, who were engaged to care for Eileen. Dr. Gelia advised me that at any time if Eileen's condition deteriorates, we could quickly transfer her to a tertiary care center. Further in-hospital studies, with a 2D echocardiography, confirmed that she had a dilated cardiomyopathy, and the pumping function had dropped to 15% (normal is 65%).

Dr. Theckedath Mathew held a family conference with us, and summarized the findings. He said that, "Eileen has a severe case of post-viral myocardiopathy, and that all necessary treatments can be accomplished at Lakeside Memorial Hospital." He was confident that she would improve quickly. She was treated with a combination of medications including Digoxin, ACE inhibitors, beta blockers, long-acting diuretics containing Aldactone, blood thinners, and Amiodarone. Eileen's condition stabilized well, and showed quick improvement. Later on she was transferred to Rochester General Hospital where cardiac catheterization confirmed that she had no evidence of obstructive atherosclerotic coronary artery disease.

A few weeks later, Eileen was all fine and well, and returned to her flower gardens to see the lilies bloom.

This case is quite unusual from at least two standpoints. The etiology of cardiac arrest is not due to acute myocardial infarction, and the bystander-initiated CPR (in this case initiated by the patient's husband) was precise and absolutely successful in reverting a potential sudden cardiac death (SCD) to a sudden cardiac death syndrome. The case cited here is an example of one the most successful bystander-initiated cardiac resuscitation I have ever come across, even though the CPR provider was not formally trained.

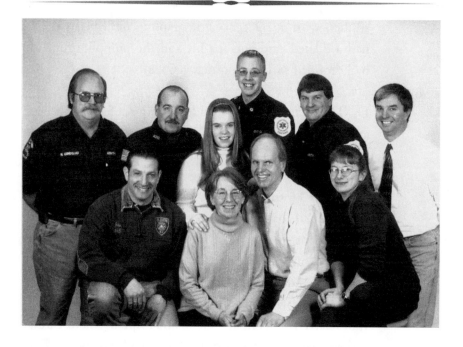

(Fig. 3) **Mrs. Eileen Bloom (Case III) and her resuscitation team, the Central Orleans Volunteer Ambulance (COVA) group.**

Pictured above: **Standing** (L – R): Nick Condoluci (COVA volunteer), Tom O'Hearn (police officer), Megan Bloom (daughter), Jeff Elsenheimer (COVA volunteer), Kent Nunnery (COVA volunteer), Eric Bradshaw (neighbor and volunteer fireman)

Sitting (L – R): Peter Sidari (volunteer fireman), Eileen Bloom, Doug Bloom, Jenna Korcz (COVA volunteer). (Missing – Keith Hale, COVA volunteer)

Blessed art thou, if substernal pain strikes you at the outset of a heart attack.

Rejoice and be glad that thou shall be rewarded with a quicker diagnosis.

Thou shall be given aspirin, clot-busters, and angioplasty most expeditiously. So, for to you I say, thou shall have a better chance of survival.

Theckedath Mathew, M.D.

Chapter Two

Acute Myocardial Infarction
Symptoms and Presentations

In my two decades of clinical observation, I can definitely say that acute myocardial infarction is the most misinterpreted and misdiagnosed clinical entity that there is, due to its diversity of symptoms and presentations.

We have to educate a community that a heart attack can occur without chest pain, and we have to reinforce our caregivers that a heart attack is possible with no startling symptoms or EKG changes.

Acute Myocardial Infarction (AMI) indeed is a deceptive disease in its presentation. Overall, not more than 70% of the afflicted group will have any kind of chest pain at all. The most popular and classical presentation of acute crushing-type of chest pain with difficulty in breathing and associated diaphoresis is mostly confined to young and middle-aged males.

This classical mode of presentation has become synonymous with the onset of an AMI, even to the extent of ignoring or even stigmatizing other modes of presentations, such as shortness of breath, nausea, vomiting, or diaphoresis, as that due to a heart attack.

Chest pain—for that matter, pain of any kind—is very poorly appreciated by diabetics because of the concomitant neuropathy in these patients. Sweating, shortness of breath, or simply not feeling well may be the sole presenting symptom of AMI in a diabetic patient.

Atypical Presentations of Heart Attack

1. Shortness of breath
2. Sweating
3. Flu-like symptoms
4. Nausea, vomiting, or indigestion
5. Neck pain
6. Jaw pain

Elderly people, due to degenerative changes in the central, peripheral and autonomic nervous system, do not usually appreciate typical chest pains of AMI. The nerve fibers that carry the pain sensation from the heart to the brain, and the brain cells that receive and interpret these sensations, could be afflicted as a part of senescence. Shortness of breath, confusion, nausea, vomiting, and diaphoresis are commonly observed symptoms of AMI in this group. I have observed that elderly people have a low threshold in presenting their symptoms, and it is not uncommon that a bystander detects color changes or a difference in breathing that will tip one off to a correct diagnosis.

Women of any age are at particular disadvantage in having little or no chest pain, in as much as 40-50% of the cases. Shortness of breath, epigastric discomfort, nausea, and diaphoresis are symptoms that are common in this group.

Shortness of breath as a presentation of AMI becomes even more of a vexing problem when it occurs in patients who already have some baseline shortness of breath from COPD (Chronic Obstructive Pulmonary Disease), severe hypertension, or obesity.

Heart attack occurring on certain locations of the heart muscle has significant difference in presenting complaints irrespective of age, sex or pre-existing conditions. Heart seizures of the inferior and back wall of the heart (diaphragmatic and posterior myocardial infarction) tend to have more of a gastrointestinal type of symptom, such as epigastric discomfort, feeling of indigestion, nausea, and vomiting. However, symptoms of diaphoresis or light-headedness (vasovagal attacks or from slow heart rate) even if very subtle, could be very, very important signals of an evolving AMI. Neck pain, jaw ache, arm pain, and posterior interscapular pain are also atypical presentations of heart attack.

There are also a few patients who develop AMI with no symptoms whatsoever, which is subsequently detected by EKG or cardiac investigations such as echocardiography, nuclear imaging, or by coronary angiography.

A patient with a "painless myocardial infarction" may arrive at an emergency room several hours later than those with pain. Thus, they have a two- to threefold increased risk of in-hospital death.

It is ideal that everyone in our community be aware of the various ways that AMI might present itself to them. After all, the patient feels the initial warning of a cardiac problem by certain signals. If you, as a patient or bystander, are unaware of the symptoms of AMI, then you may misread these signals. It is the patient or someone near the patient who is to make that FIRST CARDINAL CALL, which could lead to a prompt diagnosis and timely intervention.

In my two decades of observation as a cardiologist, I can definitely say that AMI is the most misinterpreted and misdiagnosed clinical situation by both patients as well as caregivers.

In my two decades of observation as a cardiologist, I can definitely say that Acute Myocardial Infarction is the most misinterpreted and misdiagnosed clinical situation by both patients as well as caregivers.

AMI: Clinical Presentation

AMI is one of the many ways coronary artery disease presents itself. Build up of cholesterol in the inner layer of the coronary arteries, and its eventual transformation into plaque and/or blockages is termed coronary atherosclerosis. Plaque build-ups can gradually grow within the arterial lumen, progressively decreasing the flow of blood within the blood vessel. These plaque build-ups can suddenly become unstable, leading to rupture, hemorrhage, and abrupt closure of the vessel. On the other hand, the plaque can progressively grow to the extent where it totally occludes the vessel, though the patient shows no symptoms of cardiac disease nor sustains a heart attack. This type of variation in clinical presentation is one of the many mysteries of coronary artery disease.

In general, the clinical presentation of coronary artery disease can be identified under the following categories:

Acute Coronary Syndrome
AMI presenting as sudden death
Transmural myocardial infarction
Non-Q wave or nontransmural myocardial infarction
Unstable angina

Sub-acute and Chronic Coronary Syndrome
Stable angina
Asymptomatic CAD
Walking heart attacks

AMI Presenting as Sudden Death

In a few unfortunate individuals, the initial presentation of coronary artery disease (CAD) is sudden cardiac death (SCD) during sleep. This can be considered as the adult "coronary cot death." Yet, in some others, the chest pain afflicts the individual with lightning speed and quickly deteriorates with shortness of breath, diaphoresis, syncope, and death. In these situations, an AMI will rapidly devastate the normal rhythm of the heart into chaotic, irregular, and ineffective salvos of beats (ventricular fibrillation) resulting in sudden death. Most of these individuals never even had the privilege to know that they had anything wrong with their hearts at all. In fact, sudden cardiac death is the first as well as the last presenting symptom in these individuals. Interestingly, a good many of these individuals do not even have pre-existing critical coronary stenoses. In about two-thirds of these patients with sudden cardiac arrest (SCA), the pre-existing coronary stenosis is less than 70%. At some juncture, an atherosclerotic coronary plaque becomes unstable, leading to rupture and hemorrhage, which results in total occlusion of the coronary artery.

In about 44% of men and 53% of women, sudden cardiac arrest is the first manifestation of their heart disease. In our community, sudden cardiac arrest occurs in 1 of every 10,000 residents per year. Nearly 80% of the sudden cardiac arrests occur at home, but only 60% in the presence of a witness. Survival of a sudden cardiac arrest victim is very low, particularly when it occurs at home. If SCA occurs at home, only about 8% of them are successfully resuscitated. However, if a cardiac arrest happens outside the home in the community, about 18% of them are successfully resuscitated. Timely identification of the problem, quick bystander-initiated cardiopulmonary resuscitation, and ready availability of a defibrillator are the key factors of a successful resuscitation. Quick response of paramedics and quality community hospitals with solid cardiology support are important factors in salvaging lives in this sub-group of people who are resuscitated. Roughly 250,000 lives that experience an acute myocardial infarction are lost in the field every year.

Acute Transmural Myocardial Infarction

The survival of people with acute myocardial infarction who enjoyed the benefit of early detection and timely intervention, has significantly improved over the past 10 years. From 1984-1994, the death rate from heart attack has declined by approximately 28%. Moreover, the overall severity of AMI is also decreasing. We see fewer cases of transmural myocardial infarctions, and more and more of nontransmural myocardial infarctions. We also see a trend towards quicker response of patients arriving to the ER. Yet in 1994, we lost 487,490 lives from AMI alone, making it the single most leading cause of death in the United States. This year as many as 1.5 million will sustain an AMI, and about 1/3 of them will die. However, another 500,000 patients with newly diagnosed CAD is added onto this pool, making the overall incidence of CAD somewhat unaltered. The United States has the largest block of survivors of heart attacks or people having angina—a staggering 13.7 million patients.

In about 66% of AMI victims, the cholesterol plaque in the coronary artery is 70% or less, which is non-critical. Rupture of cholesterol plaque is the fundamental pathology in acute coronary syndromes. In acute transmural (completed) myocardial infarction, a segment of the heart muscle (anterior, posterior, or diaphragmatic) is completely devoid of blood supply, resulting in muscle death. This necrotic muscle is dysfunctional and cannot partake in the pumping of blood. Therefore, in many people, the heart's pumping function deteriorates; the heart enlarges, and sometimes even forms aneurysms. This results in congestive cardiac failure, with its accompanying manifestations of shortness of breath, fluid retention, etc.

The detection of the early symptoms of AMI is the most important first step. If the patient reaches the emergency room within the first four hours of the onset of symptoms (not necessarily chest pain), we have immense possibili-

> Time is of the essence of success in salvaging life and the early golden moments of an AMI must not be wasted.

ties of helping the patient with several medications, including clot-busters (thrombolytic), antiplatelet agents, etc. A good many of the patients are also candidates for emergency angioplasty, if the hospital has such facilities. Time is of the essence for success in salvaging life, and the **early golden moments** of an AMI must not be wasted.

Nontransmural Myocardial Infarction and Unstable Angina

An erosion or rupture of an artherosclerotic plaque, activation and accumulation of platelets at the ruptured plaque site, fibrin deposition, formation of a "white clot," and coronary spasm are responsible for this entity of CAD. Here, even though the plaque rupture and the resultant physiological changes are identical to that of transmural myocardial infarction, total muscle death does not happen because of the presence of collateral circulation, and the dominating power of the body's own thrombolytic system.

Here again, timely detection of the symptoms and prompt arrival to the emergency room will help us evaluate the patient and offer the most optimal level of care. The recent availability of low-molecular weight heparins, powerful antiplatelet agents (ReoPro, Integrilin, tirofiban, Plavix), coronary balloon angioplasties, and stenting has significantly reduced the morbidity and mortality of this clinical syndrome.

Non-acute Coronary Syndromes

In stable angina, the patient indeed has quite a significant build-up of cholesterol in the coronary system, and the blockages can be up to 80% or 90%. However, the lesions are stable without inflammation, rupture, or thrombus formation. The major problem is a disparity between supply and demand. When the heart muscles demand more blood at times of increased activity, the coronary arteries are unable to deliver the amount of blood due to the blockages. This disparity in supply and demand results in ischemia of the heart muscle, which is translated as angina or anginal equivalent symptoms. Coronary spasm also plays a role in the symptomatology of stable angina.

In stable angina, the symptoms are provoked by exercise, creating a situation of supply-demand disparity. However, if the patient does not exercise on a routine basis or go to a doctor for an exercise test, this condition can go undetected, only to reappear as an acute coronary syndrome later on, with all its devastating sequelae.

Walking Heart Attack Victims

A few patients may develop relatively asymptomatic heart attacks, and therefore will not be correctly identified as AMI in a timely fashion. Elderly people, diabetics, and hypertensives with their inherent atypical presentation of symptoms belong to this group. More often than not the symptoms are limited to that of a cold or flu, or a stomach upset at the very best. In these subjects, a diagnosis of myocardial infarction is made later on from an EKG, echocardiogram, stress test, or angiogram test. The absence of classical chest pain in this group makes them vulnerable for complications of myocardial infarction and death, presumably by misinterpretation of their symptoms as something trivial. They seek medical help way too late—at times, beyond the point of no return.

> The "cardinal first call" of AMI must come from the patient or the people in close vicinity, i.e., an informed member of the community.

Now it is quite clear that AMI has a wide spectrum of presenting complaints and symptoms, confusing enough not only to patients, but to nurses and physicians as well. The initial presentation of AMI must be appreciated by the patient, and the people in the immediate surroundings. The symptoms could be as subtle as "not feeling good, some heaviness in the stomach area, feel like throwing up, or can't breathe well," etc.

Alternatively, it can also be a crushing chest pain, severe shortness of breath, diaphoresis or collapse. In any case, the "cardinal first call" of AMI must come from the patient or the people in close vicinity, i.e., an informed member of the community.

The Myth of Clot-Busters

Many people believe that those clot-busters (fibrinolytic therapy) are the panacea of modern medicine, and that everything would be fine if you received them.

It is true that clot-busters are very good and powerful medications. Timely administration of these medications can reduce the mortality of AMI by 33%. However, the vast majority of AMI patients are ineligible to receive these medications. In fact, only 20% of the patients are eligible to receive it. Late arrival to the hospital, bleeding problems, recent surgery, stroke, age above 70, severe hypertension, previous myocardial infarction, and previous bypass graft surgery are all contraindication for clot-buster administration.

Even in the best of conditions, if indeed you receive a clot-buster, the chance of a clogged artery being reopened is less than 60%.

Don't become disappointed when I tell you that even if the clogged vessel is reopened, you will still be plagued by the possibilities of acute as well as late reocclusion of those vessels, so much so that by the end of one year 70% of you will require an angiogram, angioplasty, or open-heart surgery.

Chapter Three

Cardiac Risk Factors

ardiac risk factors are the writings on the
wall. By carefully reading them, we can identify the one
who is at risk for a sudden cardiac arrest or AMI.
If an American lives up to the age of 60, he or she has a
50% chance of being afflicted by cardiovascular disease
and death.

There are several highly significant conventional cardiac risk factors such as high blood pressure, diabetes, cigarette smoking, high cholesterol, family history of coronary artery disease, overweight, and postmenopausal state that puts an individual at high risk for developing coronary artery disease and sudden cardiac death. The multiplicity of these cardiac risk factors in the same patient makes the incidence, as well as severity of the disease even higher. Based on the impact of the conventional cardiac risk factors on the pathogenesis and morbidity of CAD, they are sub-classified into major and minor risk factors:

The major cardiac risk factors have an extremely profound influence in the genesis of atherosclerotic coronary artery disease and its sequelae. The minor cardiac risk factors contribute to the risk in an additive fashion. Family history of coronary artery disease and menopause are of course non-modifiable, whereas smoking is the only cardiac risk factor that can be completely avoided. All the other cardiac risk factors have some genetic link, but can be quite remarkably modified by diet, exercise and pharmacotherapy. However, daily routine exercise (about 8 METs), remains to be the one and only intervention that will positively influence all cardiac risk factors, reversible or not.

Major

Diabetes
Smoking
Hypertension
Hypercholesterolemia
Family history
Obesity

Minor

Postmenopausal women
Men age 45 or above
Type A personality
Sedentary habits
High resting heart rate

Novel Risk Factors

Homocysteinemia
High fibrinogen level
High lipoprotein level—Lp(a)
High platelet count
Infections
Small dense low-density Lipoproteins
Thick blood (hypercoagulability)

Cardiac Risk Factor

Hypertension

ypertension is mostly an asymptomatic disease with insidious onset and progression producing permanent damage to the cardiovascular system. About 50% of the hypertensives are not treated at all.

We have made significant strides in improving the detection and management of high blood pressure, thereby reducing its complications and mortality. However, the incidence of high blood pressure remains unaltered for the past several decades. We have about 50 million Americans with high blood pressure. Hypertension is more prevalent among African-Americans and increases with age.

Hypertension is mostly an asymptomatic disease with insidious onset and progression, producing permanent damage to the cardiovascular system. Symptoms of headache or shortness of breath are late manifestations. Once high blood pressure is clinically detected, some damage has certainly occurred to the cardiovascular system. The left ventricle, the main pumping chamber of the heart, responds to long-standing hypertension by thickening and enlargement (left ventricular hypertrophy). Two types of changes occur in the arteries of a hypertensive patient. The thickening of the endothelium and the intima with the development of plaque is fundamentally the process of atherosclerosis. **ATHEROSCLEROSIS** eventually invades the intima producing sclerosis and calcification. Independent of atherosclerosis, the arteries undergo a process of **ARTERIOSCLEROSIS** with advancing age. Here, the arteries progressively lose their compliance (elasticity) and become stiff. The changes occur in the adventitia and media of the vessels where the elastic fibers are replaced by fibrous tissue and calcium. In high-risk patients, both atherosclerosis and arteriosclerosis co-exist making matters worse. However, meticulous reduction of high blood pressure certainly reduces the cardiovascular events such as myocardial infarction, stroke, and congestive heart failure.

At times it is difficult to convince the patient to accept pharmacological treatment for hypertension, particularly when the medications have some side effects, and the patient is relatively free of symptoms. The compliance to medications and maintain treatment is generally poor. That is the reason why about 50% of our hypertensives are not treated at all; about 25% are treated, but not properly controlled; and only the remaining 25% are properly managed. Salt restriction, weight reduction, exercise, and relaxation techniques have a significant impact on the management of hypertension. Above all, the awareness of this deadly disease, with its late manifestations such as stroke, heart attack, congestive heart failure, renal failure, and peripheral vascular disease must be made known to the patient at a very early stage.

Here, I shall emphasize that all hypertensives must not be viewed or treated the same way. The 6th Report of the Joint National Committee on Detection, Evaluation, and Treatment of Hypertension has made the strongest recommendation that in patients with diabetes, coronary artery disease, and renal failure any blood pressure above 130/85 mmHg must be treated. Moreover, if a patient has renal failure with proteinuria (more than 1 gram in 24 hours) the blood pressure must be kept below 125/75 mmHg.

There is a misconception among patients, as well as some physicians, that diastolic hypertension is more important than systolic hypertension. The fact is that in a truly hypertensive patient, both systolic and diastolic pressures gradually rise in a parallel fashion until the patient is 50-55 years old. At this stage, the peripheral arteries become thick and non-elastic (non-compliant). From then on, the systolic pressure could still rise while the diastolic pressure gradually falls. The fall in diastolic pressure is a function of the lack of compliance of the peripheral arteries.

This is a hypothetical example of progression of hypertension in a patient.

Patient *John Doe*

Age	BP Systolic	BP Diastolic	BP Terminology
14	118	70	Normal
24	142	92	Mild Hypertension
48	181	124	Severe Hypertension
60	218	146	Severe Hypertension
72	220	90	Hypertension
84	200	60	Isolated Systolic Hypertension

In the natural history of hypertension, "isolated systolic hypertension" (ISH) is an advanced form of the disease and therefore must be respected and managed accordingly. At the same time, one must also properly identify other causes of "ISH" due to incompetence of the aortic valve, anemia, arteriovenous fistula, beriberi, and some cases of thyrotoxicosis.

> In the natural history of hypertension, *"isolated systolic hypertension" (ISH)* is an advanced form of the disease, and therefore must be respected and managed accordingly.

White Coat Hypertension

The delineation and implication of white coat hypertension and sustained hypertension is not just clear as black and white. In fact, there is a subset of patients who have a very high blood pressure reading in a physician's office, and may have a perfectly normal blood pressure reading on ambulatory blood pressure monitoring, who can be genuinely identified as white coat hypertensive patients.

Hypertension is not an elevated blood pressure reading alone. It is a syndrome that encompasses anatomical changes in the cardiovascular system, end organ dysfunction, and allied biochemical aberrations. In these patients, the left ventricle is thicker and less compliant (LV mass index 10% above normal). They have more insulin resistance, hypertriglyceridemia, higher levels of plasma aldosterone and norepinephrine, just as in sustained hypertension. Therefore, this situation is not entirely normal.

It is my belief that white coat hypertension is an overused and oversimplified version of labile hypertension, thereby escaping the proper diagnosis and treatment of hypertension. If a person is noted to have a blood pressure of 180 or 200 in the doctor's office, and subsequently noted to have only 130 or 140 in the ambulatory setting, then that person must be identified as a hypertensive patient. Most of these patients have arteriosclerosis and are candidates to develop atherosclerosis.

Cardiac Risk Factor

Diabetes

iabetes is a real villain in the tragic human drama of coronary artery disease by convincingly masquerading its symptoms to confuse and mislead every one of the other players, even the director.

Diabetes is a disease of antiquity. The National Diabetes Data Group defines diabetes as a fasting blood sugar of 140 mg/dl or above. Over the past three decades, our diabetic population has quadrupled to about 25 million, approximately 10% of the adult American population. Of these, about 90% are adult-onset type and 10% are juvenile-onset type. Except for some pancreatic disease or injury, diabetes has a very strong genetic predisposition. The disease has an insidious onset with steady progress to permanent atherosclerosis (premature aging of the vascular system) with a predilection for heart, eyes, and kidneys.

Degenerative changes of nerve fibers in diabetics constitute the right setting for painless heart attacks in these patients. **In diabetics, a heart attack may present as sweating, weakness, shortness of breath, nausea, or vomiting.** An ill-informed patient often discounts these symptoms as "stomach flu" or "bronchitis."

> Painless heart attack is more of a norm in diabetics rather than the rule.

In the U.S. alone, 77,000 diabetics die each year from cardiovascular diseases (CAD, hypertension, and stroke) and its complications. Atherosclerosis and its complications account for 75% of mortality among diabetics.

In fact, 25% of all heart attacks in the United States occur in patients with diabetes. Diabetics in general have a poor outcome in surviving an acute myocardial infarction. They also have an increased graft occlusion rate after bypass graft surgery, and a more than average reocclusion rate following coronary angioplasty. About 50% of our adult onset diabetics are unidentified or not treated with specific medications. It is ideal to check the whole population for prevalence of diabetes, in the absence of which, individuals with a high predisposition for diabetes must be identified. They are: 1) relatives of known diabetics, 2) people with overweight, 3) mothers delivered of large babies, 4) older age group.

> About 50% of our adult-onset diabetics are unidentified or not treated with specific medications.

Since the invention of insulin in 1921, the management of diabetes has been revolutionized. Yet diabetes continues to be a major medical problem and consumes 15% of our total healthcare dollars. As the age of the U.S. population continues to increase along with the incidence of obesity, we can expect a dramatic increase of diabetes-related cardiovascular disease in the U.S.

Once you diagnose diabetes in a patient, you are about to touch the tip of an iceberg of a myriad of other problems. Diabetes almost never presents as an isolated problem in a person. There is a very high prevalence (more than 66%) of other risk factors like obesity, hypertension, and hyperlipidemia.

> Diabetics have an abnormal and aggressive inflammatory response to atherosclerosis or to other common viral or bacterial infections.

Diabetes has an abundance of other <u>non traditional risk factors</u> and <u>serum markers</u> for coronary artery disease, such as:

> High waist-to-hip ratio (Apple belly)
> High fibrinogen level
> High level of leukocyte count
> High levels of plasminogen activator inhibitor
> High levels of homocysteine
> High levels of C-reactive protein
> High Lp(a)
> Low serum albumin levels
> Microalbuminuria
> High levels of Factor VIII
> High levels of von Willebrand's factor
> Low magnesium

Based on this information, our strategy is to strive for absolute glycemic control with appropriate therapeutic agents. Lipid management with statin certainly reduces the markers of inflammation and the incidence of acute coronary syndrome. In a hyperlipidemic diabetic, the use of fibrates deserves special attention due to its effect to reduce fibrinogen. The beneficial effects of weight reduction, exercise, and smoking cessation are exceptionally useful in these patients.

The various nonspecific risk factors listed above suggest that diabetics have an abnormal and aggressive inflammatory response to atherosclerosis, or to other common viral or bacterial infections. This nonspecific inflammatory process, irrespective of its cause, leads to excessive expression of C-reactive proteins, cytokine tumor necrosis factor Alpha and fibrinogen resulting in a chain of vascular events leading to plaque rupture, hemorrhage, and thrombosis—the common denominators of acute coronary syndrome.

Aspirin and Diabetes

The time honored aspirin (Acetyl salicylic acid) champions to be the most useful pharmacological agent in the prevention of acute myocardial infarction, as well as reducing the extent and complications of this disease. Aspirin is fundamentally an anti-inflammatory agent. There is growing evidence that the cardinal precipitating cause of AMI is inflammation of the coronary arteries and atherosclerotic plaques. This inflammation leads to plaque rupture, hemorrhage and occlusion in completing the process of an acute heart attack. Thus, the role of an anti-inflammatory agent is self-explanatory.

The process of plaque inflammation and rupture are at its worst among diabetics. The daily dose of 325mg of aspirin is a must in a diabetic until and unless there is a strong contraindication. If there is a contraindication for aspirin, one should consider Clopidogrel (Plavix) 75mg once a day.

Cardiac Risk Factor

Smoking

Behold!
Wiser are those who never smoked.
Repent!

Kick that abominable habit now for thy shall be rewarded with much less chance of having heart attacks, cancer, chronic obstructive pulmonary disease, stroke, and peripheral vascular disease.

Enticing advertisements aimed at children, the social behavior of the superstars of our pop culture, the tobacco lobbyists of Washington, are all reaching the targets so well, that about 3000 more children become new smokers each day. Hail to the camel!

We have an estimated 26 million men and 23 million women who are currently smokers. Smoking takes a very high toll on human lives. From 1990-1994, on an average, 430,000 people died from smoking-related illnesses such as emphysema, cancer, and coronary artery disease. Nicotine, carbon monoxide, and tar are the major offenders inhaled with smoking. *Nicotine*, a very potent vaso-constrictor element, produces constriction of the arteries, enhances atherosclerosis, and increases the chance of thrombosis in the coronary arteries leading to heart attacks.

> Nicotine is an addictive drug, and therefore must be considered as such.

Carbon monoxide competes for the oxygen carried through the blood, thereby making this life-sustaining gas less available to the vital organs in the body. *Tar*, of course, is the major culprit for cancer. Since the mid 1960s, we have known that smoking is a major cardiac hazard, and that it increases the mortality of patients with coronary artery disease by 50%. If a person continues to smoke after a heart attack, the risk of reinfarction and death are quite markedly increased in the range of 22-50%. Continued smoking is a key factor in bypass graft atherosclerosis and thrombosis. If a patient continues to smoke after an angioplasty or coronary stenting, the restenosis rate as well as progression of disease in the unintervened vessels is high. Second-hand smoking poses substantial risk for coronary artery disease with an estimated 40,000 coronary deaths in the United States alone.

> A person known to have high risk for coronary artery disease dies 10–5 years earlier if he/she smokes.

In spite of some of the quasi-purposive measures from the United States government, and other Healthcare Maintenance Organizations, the incidence of smoking amongst young people is rapidly on the rise. Enticing advertisements aimed at children, the social behavior of the superstars of pop culture, the tobacco lobbyists of Washington are all reaching the target so well that about 3,000 more children become new smokers each day. Nicotine is an addictive drug, and therefore must be considered as such.

To live is to smoke - The Nicotine Power

A study: A couple of years back a 56-year-old man with morbid obesity (weight 380 pounds, BMI 46) came to me referred by another cardiologist for a possible repeat angiogram and intervention for recurrent angina. He was a very heavy smoker, and also had several comorbidities, including COPD, sleep apnea and bilateral below-knee amputation for poor leg circulation. He had six coronary angiograms and two angioplasties in the past. Due to extensive peripheral arterial disease, arterial access for angiogram was very difficult. I chose to go in via the axillary artery in the left armpit and performed an angiogram and deployed a stent in the right coronary artery. He was extremely thankful to me, as his previous cardiologist had told him that they would not do any more procedures on him until he stopped smoking. I politely informed him that I was also planning to join the ranks of the previous cardiologists. He virtually told me that he lives to smoke. Much more living he did not do; about three months later he succumbed to another heart attack.

Cardiac Risk Factor

High Cholesterol

he ravaging effects of hypercholesterolemia starts very early in life. We now know that even children aged 10-14, with multiple cardiac risk factors including hypercholesterolemia, have already developed coronary plaques of 40-50%. The screening for hypercholesterolemia should start at the pediatric age group.

We don't screen all of our patents for high cholesterol, let alone the young adults. Once high cholesterol is detected, adequate interventions or treatment with statins are not initiated in everyone. Once treatment is started some of the medications are not titrated to optimal levels; no wonder only a very small fraction of our patients are properly managed in this context.

High cholesterol is another major cardiac risk factor in the genesis of atherosclerosis. Low-density cholesterol is often the nidus to develop a cholesterol plaque, and will eventually clog up the coronary arteries leading to angina, myocardial infarction, or death. It is estimated that we have over 90 million adults whose cholesterol level is above 200—a situation that will warrant reevaluation and dietary modifications. However, we have over 36 million people with a cholesterol level of 240 or above—a situation that needs close attention, dietary restriction, and possibly pharmacological intervention. We clearly have about 20 million Americans who need pharmacological intervention for reducing their chances of coronary death, heart attack, and peripheral vascular disease.

Modest reduction of severe cholesterol can be achieved by strict dietary discipline. Red meat, egg, liver, bacon, cheese, lobster, and other sources of *saturated fatty acids are the major offenders* that should be curtailed or avoided.

There is a large array of cholesterol-lowering medications on the market. However, a group of drugs commonly called *statins* (simvastatin, lovastatin, pravastatin, and atorvastatin), have shown remark-

It is also encouraging and exhilarating to see that simvastatin was capable of reducing future coronary events in as much as 38% of the hypercholestrolemic population who never had clinical evidence of CAD to begin with (primary prevention).

able benefits not only in lowering cholesterol, but also in reducing the process of atherosclerosis, whose effects are later translated into lesser clinical events

In a landmark study published in 1994, popularly known as the 4S study (**The Scandinavian Simvastatin Survival Study**), when people with known CAD (marked by angina or previous MI) were treated with 20-40 mg of simvastatin, a 30-35% reduction was noted in future episodes of MI, death, or coronary bypass graft surgery.   In addition, episodes of cerebral stroke were reduced by 28%. Similar results have been reported with **pravastatin** and **atorvastatin** too.   **It is also encouraging and exhilarating to see that simvastatin and pravastatin were capable of reducing future coronary events in as much as 38% of the hypercholestrolemic population who never had clinical evidence of CAD to begin with (primary prevention).**   It must be clearly understood that the most important effect of a statin-type of cholesterol-lowering agent is to passivate an

> Of the many modalities of treatment for coronary artery disease, optimal reduction of blood cholesterol level with the help of clinically proven medications is the sole intervention that is known to arrest the progression of atherosclerosis, passivate the plaque, and even a chance to reverse this process by resorption of the plaque.

angry cholesterol plaque, thereby reducing the chance of erosion, rupture, and the subsequent chain of events.

In light of unchallengeable evidence like this, it is a crime if eligible patients are not treated with clinically proven statin agents for primary and secondary prevention of CAD.   However, it is a travesty

to see that only a meager two million people are now receiving cholesterol-lowering drugs for a disease, which is grossly under-treated.

Make it a point to take your cholesterol-lowering medications
with the evening meals, as hepatic cholesterol and triglyceride synthe-
sis occurs mostly during nighttime hours.

High Cholesterol in Women and Children

For long atherosclerosis was held synonymous to senescence.
However, we now know that aortic atherosclerosis and fatty streaks
can be seen in some children of age 5 or 6. There are numerous case
reports of heart attacks amongst teenagers. In the rare and unfortunate
scenario of Familial Homozygous Hypercholesterolemia (FHH), AMI
have been documented at an early age of 8 onwards and cardiac death
is not uncommon in the teens, twenties and thirties.

Cholesterol molecule is an integral part of cell membranes and
forms the nucleus of virtually every hormone in our body. Therefore,
interfering with the metabolism of cholesterol molecules with medications (statins) comes with a hefty load of adverse effects in growing
children and pregnant or lactating women. Pharmacological treatment with statins is not recommended in boys under the age of 19
and girls under the age of 22 with the only exception of FHH. A
woman in her childbearing years should be treated with a statin only
if she is unlikely to conceive.

Cardiac Risk Factor

Family History of

Coronary Artery Disease

$\mathcal{S}$trong family history of coronary artery disease is a very high-risk situation. Pay maximum attention to reducing all other cardiac risk factors. This is one situation where screening for novel cardiac risk factors is indicated. I have observed that in a good many of the patients with strong family history of coronary artery disease, the coronary arteries are small, at times very small, and when afflicted by atherosclerosis, it is often diffuse rather than discrete.

A strong family history of coronary artery disease with several members sustaining MI or sudden death is of utmost concern for the members of that family. Whereas family history of coronary artery disease obviously is not a reversible situation, the members of the family must be extremely careful to reduce all other cardiac risk factors, if at all possible. Genetic counseling has not been advocated in this situation.

Smoking cessation is an absolute must; low-density cholesterol is to be kept below 90 mg/dl; and blood sugar levels in diabetics are to be corrected to near-normal levels. Weight reduction and daily exercise programs are also helpful to ward off this deadly disease.

After listening to the theory of evolution by his science teacher, the boy came home and asked his mother, "Mom, is it true that we are all descendants of monkeys?" After a moment, the mother replied, "Well, my son, I am not quite sure. However, I don't know the full family history of your father."

A Case Study

I thought everything was done right. The patient was a 36-year-old man of Mediterranean descent, 62 inches tall and weighing 170 pounds. He bore a very strong family history of coronary artery disease, in that no man survived in the family beyond the age of 45; all had succumbed to heart disease and sudden cardiac death. He had a very beautiful wife and three children, physically very active, a hard worker, who never had angina or anginal equivalent symptoms.

He was bald-headed with brownish-yellow nodules of xanthelasma below both the eyelids. He had a broad chest and very thin waist with an abundance of thick and long hair all over the torso and limbs. His physical examination was normal for pulse, blood pressure, heart sounds, and the rest. A treadmill test revealed barely 1.0 mm of ST depression on the eleventh minute with no symptoms. However, he had a cholesterol level of 300 and triglycerides of 800. He was treated with aspirin, beta blockers, and a fibrate for cholesterol reduction.

I saw him two years later. He looked exactly the same, except the hairline had receded below the occiput in a crescent shape. He had complaints of increasing fatigue towards the end of the day, and his sexual life was significantly affected. His physical examination was normal and unchanged. On the treadmill he had shortness of breath from the eighth minute onwards, although the EKG still showed barely 1.0 mm ST depression, but he had profuse sweating. After the test, during the family conference, I found his wife somewhat melancholic; not at all worried about the sex, but there was this feeling in both of them that something was not right.

I performed an angiogram on him. His coronary arteries were very small with diffuse disease, where several of the major conduit vessels looked like rosary beads. A cardiac surgeon agreed to operate on him. He had a five-vessel bypass graft surgery. All went well, and he returned to his work within two months.

A year later I received a call from his wife saying that he passed away in his sleep, and that she and the family were thankful for everything I did.

On several occasions I have thought about this patient and several others with similar scenarios. There is something about a very strong family history of coronary artery disease and premature coronary death that is inexplicable, maybe fate.

Cardiac Risk Factor

Obesity

When Charles Dickens narrated the obesity-related lethargy, drowsiness, snoring, and somnolence (Pickwickian syndrome), in his most famous Pickwickian paper in 1836, it was all about great literature, good humor, money, and fame.

Today obesity is the most rapidly increasing cardiac risk factor in our community. In the 1980s, only 20% of Americans were obese, but now about 40% are obese. Lifetime health and economic consequences of obesity is staggering. One patient will cost us about $350,000.00 additional dollars for obesity-related medical problems, and lost productivity.

Obesity

Obesity is a progressively increasing health problem, spreading in epidemic proportions all across the Western world. Obesity is defined as a body mass index (BMI) of more than 30%. In the 1980s, about 20% of Americans were obese, and unfortunately, by the beginning of the new millennium, the number is now 40%.

Obesity is a major risk factor for the devel- opment of hypertension, diabetes, high triglycerides, high low-density lipid levels, and low high-density lipid levels, thereby increasing the risk of CAD. The impact of obesity on cardiac risk factors in men and women are shown in the table below. In addition, several varieties of cancers, musculoskeletal disorders, and respiratory dysfunction have been well documented.

Table I

Men Above Age 50		
Risk Factor	BMI < 25%	BMI >30% (obesity)
Hypertension	14%	39%
Diabetes	3%	6%
High LDL	16%	25%
Low HDL	9%	25%

The effect of obesity on cardiac risk factors in men.

Table II

Women Above Age 40		
Risk Factor	BMI <25%	BMI > 30% (obesity)
Hypertension	16%	42%
Diabetes	0.3%	7%
High LDL	14%	29%

The effect of obesity in woman age 40.
BMI - body mass index.

As the BMI increases above 30%, there is an exponential increase in hypertension and diabetes mellitus in both groups. The LDL cholesterol rapidly accumulates, and the good cholesterol level goes down further.

A high fat and high sugar diet predisposes a person to obesity and insulin resistance. Such diets also produce resistance to a body hormone called leptin, which is supposed to make your body slim.

Living in America, with all of its fast food luxuries, can also be considered a risk factor. For example, Japanese people living in Japan are distinctly different from the Japanese living in San Francisco, California, in terms of their body fat and cardiac risk factor profile, as shown below.

Table III

Risk Factors	Japan	San Francisco
Cholesterol	181mg/dl	228mg/dl
Body Weight	55 kg	66 kg
Heart Disease	1.3/1000/yr	3.7/1000/yr

The "risk" of living in America
The difference in serum cholesterol, body weight, and heart-disease among Japanese living in Japan and San Francisco.

The Japanese people living in San Francisco are 11 kg heavier than their counterparts in Japan, and bear the risk of high cholesterol, and three times the incidence of heart disease.

Weight reduction in an obese patient is probably the most challenging task, as it reflects and affects the personality and the dietary culture and lifestyle of the patient. For dieting to be effective, the person must change his/her lifestyle, and must be willing to do purposeful aerobic exercise. Moreover, there is a need for ongoing personal contact and reinforcement with a program supervisor. Support groups, such as Weight Watchers, are exceptionally useful.

Ever since the Phen-Fen era, physicians have great reluctance towards prescribing weight-reducing agents. I personally encourage people to consider pharmacological intervention in selected high-risk populations, as the benefits of these drugs often outweigh the side effects.

On a Personal Note

Recently I had an obese patient who came to me requesting a letter to the airlines that she will require a wide or double seat based on her medical condition, etc. Again, recently in my consulting office, a chair just split into two pieces, as a 380-pound patient sat on it for a summary discussion of the consultation. Fortunately, nothing happened to the patient. However, I am replacing those chairs with more sturdy ones.

I was unable to perform angiograms on two patients weighing more than 400 pounds within the last six months. The cardiac catheterization tables cannot handle more than 350 pounds, as it is a suspended table with one end connected to a central weight-bearing pole. Even 350 pounds is a strain to the machine, as we see the table bend, and the tail end bows down by several inches.

When it comes to invasive procedures, obese patients bear a higher risk than others. Venous and arterial access, at times, is difficult requiring multiple sticks; vascular complications are high; and deep groin bleeding is difficult to detect until late.

Obtaining an accurate blood pressure even with wider blood pressure cuffs is difficult, particularly at times of crisis. Even CPR may be ineffective in morbidly obese individuals, as the compression pressure is difficult to be translated into the thoracic cavity. Intubating a short-necked obese patient is highly challenging, even for an experienced person, and has been unsuccessful at times. Imaging these patients is challenging despite recent advances in imaging technology. Surgery-related wound infections, lung infections, deep vein thrombosis, etc., are much higher in obese subjects.

If the present trend of rapidly increasing incidence of obesity continues, it is my feeling that this disease entity alone will consume more of our resources and health care dollars than diabetes, let alone the impact of lost wages and productivity.

Consider the following in fighting Obesity

1. A change in lifestyle is a must.
2. Join a support group. (e.g., Weight Watcher, etc.).
3. Strictly avoid high fat, high sugar diets.
4. Engage in aerobic exercise.
5. Consider taking weight-reducing agents.
6. Gain a liking for fruits, vegetables, grains, and water.
7. Consider these changes and sacrifices as an investment in your future.

Obesity and Smoking

Obesity and smoking with its related medical expenses and lost wages alone will cost us 250 billion dollars every year.

Minor Cardiac Risk Factors

Postmenopausal State
Men Age 45 or Above
Type A Personality
Sedentary Habits
High Resting Pulse Rate

However, the most important step to curb the incidence of CAD in a postmenopausal woman is to bring down the cholesterol to the bare bottom levels (LDL 85 or below), and maintain it there. This step is even more important than estrogen replacement therapy.

Most of these minor cardiac risk factors serve as an adjunct for other major cardiac risk factors. An overweight postmenopausal woman who smokes has more or less the same risk as that of a male diabetic in developing coronary artery disease. With the onset of menopause women lose their estrogen-mediated cardiac protection and enter the same risk pool with men of comparable age. For long it was believed and practiced that estrogen replacement therapy (ERT) had an enormous mitigating effect on the pathogenesis, manifestations, and even complications of CAD. However, recent studies have confounded these traditional views and have confirmed that ERT not only increases the incidence of breast and uterine cancer, arterial and venous embolic disease, but also adversely affects the process of CAD. The most important step to curb the incidence of CAD in postmenopausal women is to bring down the levels of LDL to below 85 and maintain it there.

There is quite an exponential increase in the incidence of CAD and sudden death in men from around the age of 45 onwards. No specific hormonal or other factors have been elucidated yet. Maybe the process of senescence manifests around that age group with its concomitant presentation of atherosclerosis.

A middle-aged business executive, obese, always sweating, talking in a high-pitched voice, yelling, who will never let you finish a sentence in a conversation, easily getting angered with a ruddy suffused-face, working 16-18 hours a day, is a classical example of a type A personality. These types of individuals seldom go to physicians for any symptoms, self-medicate with antacids and Advil, usually have a very high pulse rate, high blood pressure, and excessive levels of catecholamines (adrenaline and other related vasoconstrictive body hormones). This type of personality, particularly when associated with other cardiac risk factors, bears a very high risk for CAD and sudden death.

Sedentary habits just decondition the whole body, more so, the cardiovascular system. The travesty of sedentary habits is that it is associated with a high pulse rate, obesity, smoking, high blood pressure, and high cholesterol. Eventually a good many of these patients will become diabetics too. Sedentary habit is an excellent catalyst for other cardiac risk factors to develop. A resting pulse rate of 84 or more is an independent cardiac risk factor for coronary artery disease and sudden death.

Perspective

The jogger treaded the park so long,
In winter, summer, fall and spring.
Fat man snoozed on the bench so long,
Feeding the birds or licking the cream.
They said "hello" or smiled at times.
Spoke none more but barring that day.
"How do you like in what you do?"
"Are you happy the way you do?"
"Of course" answered both in sync.
"I can see the world in motion,
Without jogging I don't enjoy
The frozen joints of aches and pains."
"I don't jog nor do I like
It's all aches and sprains in legs,
It is my day of watching the dolls."

Novel Cardiac Risk Factors

Homocysteine
Fibrinogen
Platelet Activity
Lipoprotien a
Small Dense LDL
Infection

*M*y cholesterol is okay. I don't smoke. I don't have diabetes or hypertension. How come I have all these blockages?

In about 50% of patients with atherosclerosis, the aforementioned conventional cardiac risk factors are absent.

"My cholesterol is okay. I don't smoke. I don't have diabetes or hypertension. How come I have all these blockages?"

This is a question I hear from my patients quite often. We have a substantial body of evidence, which suggests that there are many other factors that are responsible for premature atherosclerosis of the coronary artery. These new factors are generally called "<u>novel cardiac risk factors</u>."

To describe these novel cardiac risk factors in detail is beyond the scope of this book; therefore, they are briefly delineated below.

<u>Homocysteine</u>: High blood levels of homocysteine, an amino acid, is associated with a high incidence of CAD, peripheral arterial disease, and venous thromboembolism.

<u>Fibrinogen</u>: An association has been noted between high levels of serum fibrinogen and chronic angina leading to acute coronary syndrome. There is also a very strong correlation between high fibrinogen levels and smoking. Fibrinogen is pro-atherogenic by increasing blood viscosity, coagulability, smooth muscle proliferation, and platelet aggregation. Poor breakdown of fibrinogen (impaired fibrinolysis) can also increase the risk.

<u>Platelet Activity</u>: Platelets play a pivotal role in the rupture of atherosclerotic plaque, which leads to acute coronary syndrome. People with high platelet counts and high platelet aggregation are more prone to acute coronary syndrome. However, there are several

steps one could undertake to reduce platelet aggregation, such as taking an aspirin a day, bringing down the blood sugar to a more optimal level, and increasing the intake of omega-3 fatty acids (commonly found in fish oils), and vitamin E. A diet with a high ratio of polyunsaturated fat to saturated fat, and the modest consumption of red wine are also useful.

Lipoprotein a—Lp(a): Lp(little)a, as conventionally called, belongs to a subset of low-density lipoproteins (bad cholesterol) associated with an increased risk of premature coronary artery disease. It has a strong heritable component, and therefore runs in families. Lp(a) also has a predisposition to run high in African-American populations. Lp(a) is considered to be an independent risk factor for CAD in Caucasian men with hypercholesterolemia.

There are some patients with high levels of LDL taking cholesterol-reducing medications, yet their LDL values remain very high. These patients are potential carriers of high levels of Lp(a).

Lp(a) is highly atherogenic and thrombogenic, and promotes human vascular smooth muscle cell proliferation. These patients are

In the Lp(a) high risk population, high levels of the lipoprotein are already present at infancy and are maintained throughout life. People who do not have conventional cardiac risk factors, and are afflicted by CAD, may be harboring high levels of Lp(a), and therefore must be screened for this type of cholesterol.

also prone to rapid restenosis after coronary angioplasty or stenting, decreased patency after coronary thrombolysis, and in some subjects produce rapid progression of CAD to diffuse coronary vasculopathy. As it stands now, there are no pharmacological agents that would satisfactorily reduce this Lp(a) level. However, substantial reduction of LDL, estrogen replacement therapy, nicotinic acid, Gemfibrozil, fish oil, and modest consumption of alcohol are all somewhat helpful in reducing the serum Lp(a) levels.

<u>Small-dense LDL and atherogenic dyslipidemia</u>: Atherogenic dyslipidemia is a malignant form of aggressive diffuse inflammatory atherosclerosis with a cluster of factors including high levels of small-dense LDL, normal levels of LDL, normal or low levels of HDL, high triglycerides, and insulin resistance. The small-dense LDL enters the vascular lining membrane (endothelium) very quickly, becomes oxidized, and evokes an aggressive process of inflammatory atherosclerosis. Treatment with Niacin appears to be very promising in this subset of dyslipidemia.

<u>Infections</u>: Chlamydia Pneumoniae, H. pylori, and Epstein-Barr virus have been attributed to inflammation of atherosclerotic plaque in coronary arteries leading to rupture, hemorrhage, and resultant heart attacks. The issue of Chlamydia Pneumoniae infection is briefly described elsewhere in this book.

Inflammation of atherosclerotic plaques, infectious or not, produces local rise of temperature in the plaques and liberates C-Reactive Proteins (CRP) into the blood. These CRP activities can be assessed by simple bedside blood tests, whereby we can screen out high-risk patients for appropriate interventions.

Chapter Four

Individual Responsibilities

Your health is your responsibility. You have to service and maintain your health...You even will have to identify the early warning signals of heart attack... You must be familiar with the atypical presentation of heart attack...At that ultimate moment of crisis—you are on your own...Having good health insurance or a great doctor isn't good enough.

69

Individual Responsibilities

Maintenance of your health is fundamentally your responsibility. The old diction "prevention is better than cure" itself is paradoxical in the case of CVD as it is not a curable disease once established. Modification of the various cardiac risk factors, and utilization of all high tech modalities of treatment can certainly alter the course of the disease problem in your favor, but certainly not curative.

Today if an American lives up to the age of 60 or above, he or she has a 50/50 chance of dying from Cardiovascular Disease.

Therefore, it is all the more important that you be aware of the various cardiac risk factors that could lead to premature atherosclerosis of the coronary arteries, and take stepwise measures to modify the risk factors to the best of your ability. However, even with the best of your efforts, CAD will still afflict individuals, and the toll on human life will still continue no matter what, but hopefully to a lesser extent. **Today if an American lives up to the age of 60 or above, he or she has a 50/50 chance of dying from cardiovascular disease.** Needless to say, this is an issue very close to home.

Typical and atypical presentations of coronary artery disease must be made very well known to the individual, particularly those at high risk. Chest pain is not always a must for heart attack. The older the individual is, the more atypical the presentation will be. An epigastric discomfort in a 25-year-old man with no cardiac risk factors could be a case of mild indigestion; however, the same symptoms in a 55-year-old diabetic who smokes might signal the onset of a heart attack. In a high-risk individual for coronary artery disease, symptoms of fatigue, sweating, indigestion, and shortness of breath must be viewed with caution.

Individual Responsibility—A Personal Agenda

Every individual must take the issue of CAD quite seriously and make an attempt to *learn more* about it.

An individual must *be fully aware* of the major and minor cardiac risk factors that put him/her at high risk for coronary artery disease.

Individuals must take every step to *modify the risk factors* so that the chance and severity of CAD is reduced.

Be aware of the typical as well as the *atypical presentation of CAD*, particularly people at high risk for CAD.

In suspected situations of heart seizure, make *the first cardinal call* as early as possible so that a disastrous situation can be avoided; every second counts, they are the golden moments.

In high risk patients with typical or atypical complaints of chest discomfort, *chew a SOLUBLE ASPIRIN as early as you can*. If a soluble aspirin is not available, take any type of aspirin, but you must chew first and then swallow. You must always keep Nitroglycerin and soluble aspirin within easy reach.

Preferably every adult should know the technique of ***Cardio Pulmonary Resuscitation (CPR)*** and must have periodic training and recertification. Certainly, the family members or co-inhabitants of a CAD patient must have proficiency in CPR.

If an individual feels lightheaded, he or she must lie down, preferably with the legs elevated and try to practice ***rhythmic coughing*** of about 40-50 per minute. Coughing is considered to be ***an internal CPR.***

The availability of a ***Defibrillator*** in the house of a high-risk cardiac patient is encouraged. There must be someone in the house who will have the expertise and presence of mind to use the equipment correctly.

<u>A poet and philosopher</u>

"The art of medicine consists of trying to amuse the patient while nature takes its own course."
Voltaire
(Paris, 1694-1778)

nstead of noble men, let us have noble villages of men. If it is necessary, omit one bridge over the river, go around a little there, and throw one arch at least over the darker gulf of ignorance which surrounds us.

**Henry David Thoreau
(1817-1862)**

Chapter Five

Community Agenda

The sound health of an individual reflects on the well-being of the community...ill health of an individual from any which reason will affect you quite directly by depleting the community resources, hospital resources, higher premiums on health insurances, taxes, and the related whole nine-yards of it.

AMI is so much a problem of the community as much as it is that of an individual. Although we as a nation are spending $160 billion every year towards the case management of CVD, there is no single agency in the community with defined responsibilities of tackling the problem overall at a community level.

> The PCP's do not have enough time to spend, incentives or remuneration to undertake a community agenda as elaborate as we are discussing here.

Primary care physicians (PCP) as a group do a fair amount of work in terms of patient education and risk factor modification; however, the service is highly limited to the patients who are registered with them. The PCP's do not have enough time to spend, incentives or remuneration to undertake a community agenda as elaborate as we are discussing here.

In this HMO-infested environment, hospitals as a whole are preoccupied with the thought of staying afloat, focusing all their energy in consolidations, mergers, and maintaining or expanding their market share. They are even firing hospital employees who are "non-essential" to direct patient care, to maintain the bottom line of the accounting book in the black.

> The HMOs would like to see cardiovascular diseases completely wiped out at no cost to them.

The HMOs would like to see cardiovascular diseases completely wiped out at no cost to them. It is no secret that their sole concentration is to trim and slim the health care delivery so that dollars are saved at the end of the day. HMOs have done an outstanding job in curtailing the choices of the patient for M.D. visits, specialist visits, brand of medications, and even several procedures. Most HMOs even demand a "pre-approval" for a patient to visit the ER, even if the complaint is chest pain. It is obvious to me that in the present environment, the HMOs will not move their little finger or shell out a dime toward developing a community aware of its CV problems.

> It is obvious to me that in the present environment, the HMOs will not move their little finger or shell out a dime toward developing a community aware of its CV problems.

Schools are an excellent point of entry for health education, to increase the awareness of CAD, its sequelae, and its impact on the community. However, most of the efforts on public health education of school districts are centered on teaching the kids how to use a condom properly. Moreover, new sets of issues like prayers, display of Ten Commandments, gun violence, etc., usually fills the agenda of school board meetings leaving CAD on the backburner.

Voluntary organizations, such as the AHA, through its local chapters, have made some effort to heighten the awareness of CVD in the community. They also have distributed various types of pamphlets, organized CPR classes, and even Heart Balls to raise awareness. Though their efforts are well-intended, they are fundamentally off target, too little, and at times seem just decorative. Volunteerism itself has its own limitations.

The media, in general, inclusive of radio, television, and movies has been historically insensitive to health care issues except when it comes to medical breakthroughs or sensational news. The discussion of public health issues in newspapers, radio, or television does not improve their circulation, the number of advertising clients, or Nielson ratings; and therefore just does not interest them. Moreover, media campaigns by radio, television, and newspapers have not been found to be useful in increasing the awareness of coronary artery disease, or the atypical presentation of acute myocardial infarction. Although the general reaction of such campaigns are very positive; the details of the messages are neither transmitted precisely nor retained well by the public. The brevity of the message and stereotypical presentations can even be misleading.

From the aforementioned discussions, it is obvious that there is no agency or organization that is responsible for the health maintenance of our community except some state-mandated emergency care through our hospitals. There are neither federal, state or local funds appropriated, nor responsibilities delegated towards this cause. In essence, health maintenance as an agenda is a responsibility left to each individual.

An individual or a family of several individuals makes up a community unit. The health and prosperity of a community depends on the well being of its individual units.

Management of an individual's health is considered his own business, and mismanagement is a fundamental right that cannot be regulated. As a society, we have successfully regulated several aspects of social behavior such as speed limits on highways and byways, instituting seatbelts, checking alcohol levels while driving, etc., in the

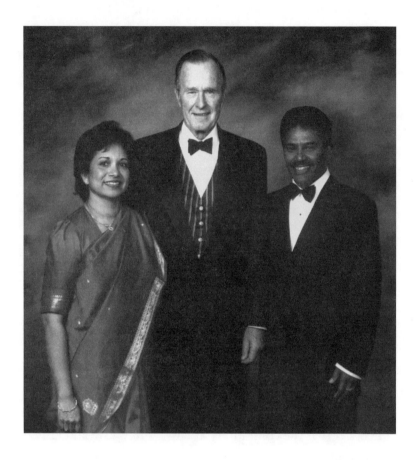

(**Fig. 4**)   President George W. Bush visited Lakeside Memorial Hospital in November 1997.

Pictured above: Susan Mathew, President Bush, and the author, Dr. Theckedath Mathew.

A Role Model Hospital

Lakeside Memorial Hospital in Brockport, upstate New York, is a small community hospital with 95 inpatient beds. This hospital has a motto, "Quality Care Close to Home." This hospital has a Family Wellness Center. This hospital has a philosophy of community involvement, and has a community agenda for acute myocardial infarctions.

I believe Lakeside Memorial Hospital with all its community outreach programs is (should be) a role model for all small community hospitals in the United States. Several national and international dignitaries have visited and complimented this hospital for its outstanding work. President Gerald Ford, President George Bush, General Norman Schwarzkopf, General Colin Powell, and British Prime Minister John Major were among those dignitaries.

There is a need for a campaign aimed at increasing the public awareness of CAD and sudden cardiac arrest (SCA). I believe a community agenda should include at least the following points for discussion, education, and implementation:

1. <u>Heart Awareness Program</u>:

It is ideal that every community hospital has a Family Wellness Center. Volunteers at no extra cost for hospitals can effectively run these Wellness Centers. "Heart awareness" should be an important agenda of these centers.

The first set of people to be focused on are the survivors of heart attacks and people with established heart diseases—i.e., the CV patient pool (CVPP). In our community, 5% of the population belongs to the cardiovascular patient pool. In a community of 200,000, there will be about 1,000 individuals who are either survivors of a heart attack or having established cardiovascular problems (CVPP). Our goal is to assemble this group once in every two months or so to a place of easy approach for a heart awareness evening. The most difficult step is to get these people under one roof at the same time. Once they are there, the remaining portion of the agenda is a piece of cake. Some of the essential components of such a town meeting should include the following:

A health care person can present and discuss cases of acute myocardial infarction, promptly identified by the patient or the family that led to a timely intervention and good outcome. But more importantly, focus at least on one case where an atypical presentation of an acute myocardial infarction (obviously without chest pain) that led to delayed reporting to the hospital and eventually a poor outcome.

Encourage the members to discuss their own experience for the benefit of others, highlighting the merits and pitfalls in the overall case management.

The aforementioned Case III in this book is an excellent case to be discussed in such situations.

In a cardiac crisis, at that moment of truth, you are on your own; you are either the patient or an immediate witness to a cardiac crisis. There are a few immediate steps you should be doing automatically, e.g., taking an aspirin, calling 911, initiate CPR (remember the steps), rhythmic coughing if needed, etc. There is an absolute need for these individuals to be trained for those moments of crisis. In our meetings, such cardiac crisis situations can be enacted by our members to make it a more interesting and meaningful educational experience.

Brief interesting didactic lectures on various subjects with a lot of emphasis on the mysteries of acute myocardial infarction, particularly in atypical presentations.

Teaching lessons on how to record heart rate and blood pressure properly, and how to properly keep a record of weight, blood pressure, and pulse rate with entries of the patient's symptoms into a journal.

To enumerate my vision on the activities of a heart awareness program is simply beyond the scope of this book. However, through the cardiac patients, we can gain access into the immediate relatives of the patients, and eventually to the community at large.

2. <u>Automated 911 System</u>:

When an individual seeks help via the 911 system, there should not be any protracted discussions about the location or the route to reach there. There are instances when a panicked 911 caller cannot even identify the street, abode, or telephone number correctly. The community should update the 911 system, so that the telephone operator should instantly know the town, street, house, or apartment where the call originated. However, the widespread use of cell phones will contrast a problem in the above context.

3. <u>CPR Skills</u>:

Ideally, every able-bodied citizen should be able to initiate CPR. To achieve that goal a lot of efforts and resources are needed. With all its merits and limitations, we still have to depend on volunteers.

The steps of CPR are simple, but difficult to remember by a layperson without periodic updating; also the guidelines change occasionally. Moreover, when it comes to real life settings, you need a lot more training and practice to successfully execute these steps.

The heart awareness programs are excellent stages to rehearse the final scene of the human drama—the CPR.

4. <u>Defibrillators</u>:

An immediate bystander-initiated CPR and the availability of a defibrillator within three minutes are the two most essential factors in the successful resuscitation of a cardiac arrest victim. The ready availability of a defibrillator just cannot be overemphasized. I believe the following organizations, individuals, or places should have defibrillators and personnel trained in its use:

a. All EMTs.

b. All firefighters.

c. All police cars.

d. All public places: hotels, restaurants, shops, malls, government buildings, court houses, schools, colleges, ships, planes, trains, buses, etc.

e. The home of a patient at high risk for sudden cardiac arrest.

N.B. The role of defibrillators is described in the succeeding pages.

5. <u>High Risk – Special Education</u>:

The people at very high risk for sudden cardiac arrest and other acute cardiac events can be identified as described in the succeeding pages.

Cardiac arrest when it occurs to someone dear to you, is a frightening moment of truth with all its suspense, fear, uncertainty, and helplessness that may transcend individuals into a state of freeze, with which they become motionless and at times accommodate themselves into a state of fainting. It is not at all uncommon to find two equally afflicted individuals in the same abode where one just is unable to help the other in such demanding situations. In such instances, there needs to be a mechanism to seek help by means of an alarm monitor or a programmed 911 call. In any case, the cohabitant of a high-risk cardiac patient needs special attention and training to cope with an adverse situation. Heart awareness meetings are ideal platforms for such activities.

Chapter Six

Syncope – The Role of Coughing
The Role of Defibrillators
The Mystery of Hypertension
Sudden Cardiac Death Syndrome

1. Syncope: The Role of Coughing

In the early phase of an acute myocardial infarction, some patients develop lightheadedness, blurring of vision, diaphoresis, and fainting. An observer usually finds that the color changes on the patient into an ashen-gray, and the body feels cold and clammy. With this presentation, some patients lose consciousness and slump to the floor in frank syncope. This situation is usually due to vasovagal attacks that lead to neurocardiac syncope or advanced heart block with severe bradycardia. Here, the pain or injury in the heart muscle evokes a peculiar neural reaction mediated through the tenth cranial nerve (the vagus nerve), resulting in bradycardia and severe vasodilatation. The patient experiences a precipitous drop in blood pressure, heart rate, or both leading to suboptimal perfusion of the vital organs particularly the brain and the heart, resulting in neurocardiac syncope.

This type of syncope, at times, is lethal if not timely intervened. An informed bystander must place the patient flat on a bed or floor without any pillows and must elevate both legs at 45 degrees. Then he/she must advise the patient to cough continuously at a rate of 40-50 coughs per minute. A good cough produces a strong contraction of the diaphragm and the intercostal muscles, resulting in sudden elevation of intrathoracic pressure, as much as 60-80 mmHg (**Fig. 5**). This cough-assisted increase in the intrathoracic pressure is also reflected in the central aortic blood pressure (the most vital measure of blood pressure), resulting in better perfusion of the brain and heart. In fact, by coughing you are increasing the blood pressure of a hypotensive patient to achieve better levels of perfusion pressures. Coughing is an internal CPR. In many instances, this maneuver alone will bring a patient out of presyncope with restoration of color, heart rate, and blood pressure. However, these maneuvers must be considered only as a first aid and should not be substituted for other important steps, such as calling 911, etc.

Case Study

Cough - An Internal CPR

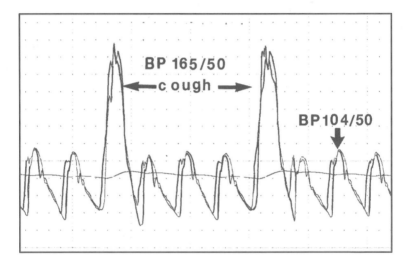

(**Fig. 5**)   The figure above shows arterial pressure tracings and EKG tracings of an 80-year-old man while undergoing a left heart catheterization. The initial blood pressure was 180/94. A left coronary angiogram revealed multiple 90-95% blockages. During angiogram, the patient developed chest pain, shortness of breath, and diaphoresis. The systolic blood pressure dropped from 180 to 100 mmHg. The patient was asked to cough. With each cough, the central aortic and peripheral blood pressure increased to 165 mmHg, thereby improving critical perfusion to the brain and other vital organs. With additional medications, the patient's blood pressure steadily improved and settled at 170/90.

When a patient is fainting with a cardiac cause such as slow heart rate, vasovagal attacks, or even ventricular fibrillation, the blood pressure precipitously drops resulting in poor or no perfusion to vital organs, particularly the brain and heart. In the very early phase of this critical moment, if the patient can cough, the central aortic pressure will instantaneously rise resulting in better perfusion of the brain, and can be lifesaving. However, the patient must be told to do so before completely passing out.

I herewith denote an incident that happened to me about a year ago. I am physically very healthy and active. Except for mild hypercholesterolemia and occasional discomfort from bursitis on my left shoulder, I have never had any other medical problems. I neither have any significant cardiac risk factors nor evidence of coronary artery disease.

I went to my physician's office for a steroid injection on my left shoulder for bursitis. The initial vitals read as a pulse rate of 72 and blood pressure of 124/70. Soon after the injection I felt warm and broke into a heavy sweat. I felt somewhat lightheaded, "weightless," and things around me were just foggy. I felt for my pulse and there was none. I started to cough immediately and continuously; I lay down on the couch, and crouched my legs with my knees up. Within a few seconds, I felt "life" gushing into my brain and things started to clear up.

What I felt was a classical episode of vasovagal attack. What I did was exactly what had to be done, and needs to be done in similar situations. Such situations are not at all uncommon in daily life, particularly secondary to a pain reaction from trauma, needle injections, or pain from any of the visceral organs.   It is my feeling that many of the "deaths on the dentist's chair" are secondary to vasovagal attacks, and its poor management by ignorant caregivers.

A Hunter's Attack

Steady, the hunter strung his bow,
ready to fell the flurrying doe.
"Hss, hss" sprang a noise from his right,
the hunter turned in frantic fright.

Sighted the raging spitting snake,
fell to the ground the hunter faint.
Sensing the hunter surely dead,
the sighing serpent hurriedly fled.

Awoke in foggy the hunter wondered,
what a Vaso-Vagal an Attack.

Ajay Mathew, NYU
two and zero zero two

2. The Role of Defibrillators

The perception that cardiac arrest is an event that can only be managed by a physician in a hospital must change. Early bystander-initiated CPR and rapid defibrillation are the two major contributions in salvaging lives in a sudden cardiac arrest situation. Sudden cardiac arrest happens anywhere in the community, and therefore the citizenry at large must be informed and equipped to provide early bystander-initiated CPR. A lot more people in the community other than physicians, nurses, or paramedics must know the technique of CPR. It is most ideal that every able adolescent and adult be proficient in the technique of CPR. Next to that, all police officers, firefighters, security guards, teachers, air flight crew, health aides and other volunteers must be taught in the skill of CPR with periodic updates and reviews. Spouses and significant others of high-risk cardiac patients must be encouraged to take CPR courses.

CPR can provide a temporizing first step in the sudden cardiac arrest victim. The most significant lifesaving measure comes from the defibrillation. With very rare exception, sudden cardiac arrest results from ventricular fibrillation (salvos of ineffective chaotic cardiac electrical activity). If the situation is allowed to continue over 4 minutes, irreversible brain death is almost sure to occur. Many communities have tried to reach the victim within a period of 3-5 minutes with a team such as EMTs and paramedics equipped with defibrillators. In the United States, only about 40% of the EMTs are actually equipped with automatic external defibrillators. However, our goal of a community equipped with adequate numbers of defibrillators and individuals who know how to use them continues to be a Utopian ideal, and the life loss from sudden cardiac arrest of about 1,000 per day continues unabated. In large urban and rural communities, the paramedics can't reach the location in time, due to heavy traffic or poor route directions.

93

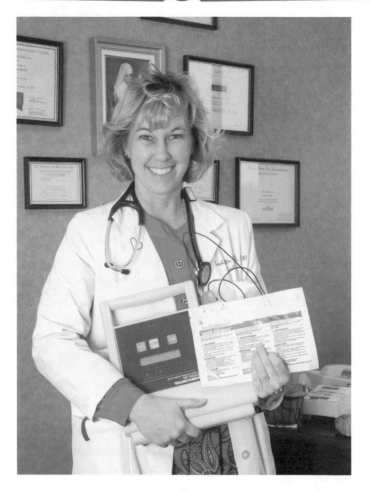

(**Fig. 6**) Terri Folts, N.P. with an automatic defibrillator.

Ideally, a portable automatic defibrillator must be available to every citizen within about four minutes from the outset of a disastrous cardiac arrest. Implementing an aggressive defibrillation strategy with the use of AEDs (automatic external defibrillators) has shown significant improvement in the survival of sudden cardiac arrest   victims. These automatic external defibrillators are small, portable, and easy to use. The use of AEDs can be safely integrated into the currently existing public safety systems such as EMTs, police,   firefighters, and the first aid responders who have a duty to respond to a sudden death event.

Air Force One and several other commercial airlines currently have AEDs with trained personnel in case of cardiac emergencies. Barring several legal and ethical issues, the prospectus of having AEDs in public places such as office buildings, hotels, cruise ships, shopping malls, retirement communities, airports, public buildings, and apartment buildings are real possibilities in the near future.

Prompt defibrillation remains the cornerstone of survival of an out-of-hospital cardiac arrest. In New York State, in 1994, only 26 out of 2329 (9%) sudden cardiac arrest victims survived when SCA was out-of-hospital. However, in Rochester, Minnesota, when police vehicles were equipped with portable defibrillation devices, 21 out of the 44 victims (50%) attended by the police survived with the help of defibrillators. The usefulness of defibrillators in the field is self-explanatory.

3. The Mystery of Hypertension

It is my belief that an accurate measurement of blood pressure is a difficult physical finding to elicit accurately. There are many reasons why it is so:

1. Blood pressure maintenance is a highly dynamic process with diurnal variations and significant fluctuations in response to neurocardiac reflexes such as anxiety, fear, a strange environment, etc. Therefore, blood pressure can vary as much as 60-80 mmHg or more at very short intervals.

2. Most hypertensive patients are on some kind of diuretics or vasodilators. Marked fluctuations in blood pressure are observed based on pharmacokinetics of the drug. For example, a hypertensive patient had a blood pressure of 190/110 at 7:00 a.m. recorded by an electronic device. Following 40 mg of p.o. Lasix and 10 mg of Vasotec, at about 10 a.m. the blood pressure recorded was 130/100 in the primary care physician's office. I saw the same patient at about 2:00 p.m. for a pacer check and cardiac follow-up visit. Her blood pressure was 230/140, 220/135, and 214/135 on three measurements. The quick natriuresis and volume depletion from Lasix, the effect of Vasotec, and the blood pressure measuring techniques are responsible for these wide blood pressure variations. Very potent short-acting loop diuretics are not ideal for long-term treatment of hypertension. One must use a low dose, long-acting diuretic for slow sustained natriuresis, and prolonged blood pressure control.

3. Elderly hypertensive patients exhibit remarkable blood pressure variations after meals, particularly breakfast. A significant drop

in systolic blood pressure, as much as 50-60 mmHg, can be seen following a heavy breakfast secondary to splanchnic blood pooling and the relatively poor sympathetic tone early in the morning.

4. Arteriosclerosis seen in the elderly and the resultant stiffness of the vessel makes cuff blood pressure measurement inaccurate.

5. One must use a high quality, well-calibrated blood pressure cuff suited to the arm size and high fidelity stethoscope to measure blood pressure. In an elderly person with arteriosclerosis, it is difficult to occlude the brachial artery circulation by applying cuff pressure. Once it is finally occluded, and then gradually released for measuring blood pressure, the initial 30-40 mm of systolic blood pressures are often missed, as they are very faint and inaudible for an inexperienced caregiver.

6. Postural hypotension is not at all uncommon in elderly people. A blood pressure recorded in recumbent position, and that measured while sitting or standing, can have significant differences. This difference is often not identified or recorded, resulting in disparity of blood pressure measurement from one office to the other.

7. Subclavian and innominate artery stenosis is also not uncommon in the elderly population. There is a common tradition of measuring blood pressure only on the right arm. This tradition makes the blood pressure measurements susceptible to inaccuracies created by brachial artery stenosis. Therefore, I recommend blood pressure measurements on both arms.

Case Study

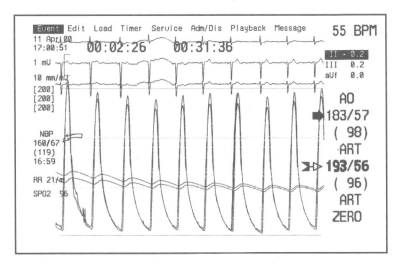

(**Fig.** 7) The EKG and pressure tracings in the picture are obtained from an 85-year-old patient with unstable angina who underwent a cath-plasty procedure. The blood pressure during the pre-cath evaluation was 155/60, 165/60, etc., suggesting mild isolated systolic hypertension.

The picture shows three sets of blood pressures measured simultaneously. The solid arrow shows blood pressure of 183/57 is a **direct measurement** from the central aorta. The flagged arrow of blood pressure 193/56 is a **direct measurement** from the femoral artery. The open arrow with blood pressure of 160/67 is a simultaneous digital blood pressure reading from the left arm by a blood pressure cuff.

The disparities in the blood pressure readings are quite obvious. This patient certainly did not have subclavian artery stenosis (blood vessel to the upper limb), and the blood pressure on the right arm was identical to the one on the left arm. Obviously, the blood pressure measured by the cuff is very, very low and wrong. Ironically, cuff blood pressure is the one we always use for clinical assessments and pharmacological interventions.

In my overall clinical assessment, high blood pressure is more often underestimated than not. Measuring blood pressure in a patient with arteriosclerosis is a difficult task loaded with possibilities of errors. Our health care providers must be aware of the several variables that I have mentioned above.

Moreover, high blood pressure is mostly an asymptomatic disease. The side effects from medications are often unpleasant and inconvenient. The patients themselves love to hear that their blood pressure is normal. Some patients even have become very upset having noted this "grossly abnormal blood pressure" in my office, and will keep on justifying the blood pressure they saw at the nearby supermarket a few weeks back. The mystery of hypertension!

4. Sudden Cardiac Death Syndrome

Before I define sudden cardiac death syndrome, I would like you to be familiar with the term of sudden cardiac arrest and sudden cardiac death.

Sudden Cardiac Arrest (SCA)

Sudden cardiac arrest is defined as the sudden and unexpected arrest of cardiac pumping function, usually initiated by a cardiac arrhythmia—(ventricular fibrillation)—that rapidly deteriorates into a cardiac standstill. The patient faints and will be pulseless. This condition is fatal if not successfully intervened and resuscitated.

CAD is the most common cause of sudden cardiac arrest. Sudden rupture of a non-occlusive atherosclerotic plaque leading to hemorrhage, thrombosis, and occlusion of the coronary artery is the most common cause. It is startling to learn that in 44% of the men and 53% of the women victims of sudden cardiac arrest, SCA is the first manifestation of CAD.

Sudden cardiac arrest usually occurs at home, most of them are unwitnessed, and the person dies. Even a witnessed sudden cardiac arrest at home bears a very poor immediate survival of 8%. However, a witnessed sudden cardiac arrest outside the home has a better chance of immediate survival of 18%, still very poor.

Sudden Cardiac Death (SCD)

Sudden cardiac death is defined as the sudden and unexpected arrest of cardiac pumping function, usually initiated by a cardiac arrhythmia—(ventricular fibrillation)—that rapidly deteriorates into cardiac standstill and death.

Sudden Cardiac Death Syndrome (SCDS)

Survivors of sudden cardiac arrest are defined as people who have sustained a sudden cardiac death syndrome. The patient in Case III described in the previous pages is a typical example of someone who has sustained a sudden cardiac death syndrome.

Case Study

I herewith enclose briefly the story of Mr. Carmine Ciccarone who is a survivor of sudden cardiac death syndrome... It was in the fall of 1984 that I met Carmine Ciccarone in the Emergency Room at Rochester General Hospital. His primary care physician alerted me that Carmine was on the way to the Emergency Room in full-blown cardiac arrest receiving CPR. Upon arrival to the Emergency Room, Carmine's life was sustained by CPR with intravenous fluids and external cardiac compression. He was immediately intubated and put on an assisted-breathing system. He did not have any intrinsic heartbeats, except a coarse ventricular tachycardia. In addition to the CPR management and defibrillation, I placed a temporary pacemaker into the apex of his right ventricle via the left subclavian vein. At this point, Carmine had a totally pacemaker-dependent rhythm with the blood pressure in the range of 70-80 mmHg. Even though he received all types of management commensurate with the

ACLS II protocol, he did not respond with any intrinsic heart rate.

For the next twelve hours, he still did not have any intrinsic pulse rate, except rare ventricular escape beats. However, with the pacemaker he maintained a blood pressure in the range of 90-100 mmHg systolic. He was dependent on a respirator, and his pupils were moderately dilated and totally unresponsive. At around midnight, the pacemaker started some sensing abnormalities. At that point, I inserted a second temporary pacemaker via the right femoral vein into the right ventricle, and started pacing with the second pacemaker. His situation was quite critical and the family was cautioned to expect the worse.

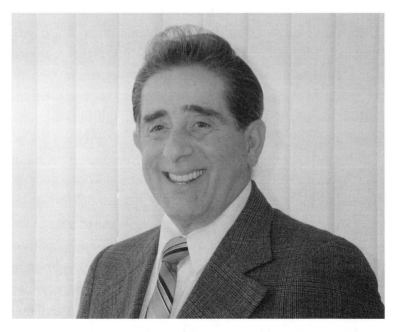

(**Fig. 8**) Carmine Ciccarone in December 2000.

After approximately 48 hours, Carmine responded with some P waves and occasional junctional QRS complexes. This intrinsic process was supported by administration of atropine and other supportive measures. Within a few hours, he developed a normal sinus rhythm of his own. The pacemakers were subsequently withdrawn. His blood pressure improved to 120 mmHg.

His central nervous system function gradually regained over a period of 3-4 days. He certainly had evidence of anoxic encephalopathy during this hospitalization.

Subsequently, he had an angiogram and angioplasty of the right coronary artery. Carmine Ciccarone is a survivor of sudden cardiac arrest, and he indeed sustained a sudden cardiac death syndrome.

The dismal immediate survival rates of sudden cardiac arrest victims at home deserve some reflections here. It is my feeling that until and unless the cohabitant of the victim is tutored and coached, that individual may not be able to handle this crisis successfully. A few of them freeze with emotions and remain motionless, not even able to handle a 911 call. Yet, some others become panicky, inappropriately wasting the golden moments of a real resuscitation. Though rare, the witnesses themselves can faint and sustain a sudden cardiac arrest. Only very, very few of the cohabitants can stand up to that moment of crisis and initiate steps to save that life. Hence, there is an absolute need for a crisis management coaching program, at least for the cohabitants of patients who are at high risk for sudden cardiac arrest. I have some suggestions:

1. A single touch automated dialing of 911 with a prere-corded message of a cardiac event seeking immediate help

with clear directions to the location of the event should be programmed into the telephone operator. There has to be some discussion and agreement regarding the format of this message and willingness of the telephone exchanges to act on a recorded message.

2. The bystander should initiate CPR immediately.

3. The time is now ripe to consider home defibrillators, at least in high-risk situations.

The present day automated defibrillators are lightweight and easy to hook up to the patient. The machine will speak to you, it will determine the rhythm correctly, and will discharge the right amount of currents for that abnormal rhythm. However, the cohabitant must be familiarized with the defibrillator before it can be effectively used.

What about the majority of the population (0.1% to 0.15%) who are asymptomatic in whom sudden cardiac arrest is the first presentation of coronary artery disease? Is it practical and cost-effective that all dwellings be equipped with an automatic defibrillator? That all the citizenry be familiarized with this equipment? The question is more philosophical than financial or practical.

Heart Rate Index and Sudden Cardiac Death

A high resting heart rate (more than 84 beats per minute) is an independent cardiac risk factor for mortality in patients with acute myocardial infarction, hypertension, and the elderly with heart diseases. This is thought to be secondary to abnormalities in the autonomic nervous system with increased sympathetic activity, reduced vagal activity, or a combination of both. This situation lowers the threshold for ventricular fibrillation and sudden cardiac death.

Another important observation is *chronotropic incompetence* (failure to achieve 85% of age-adjusted predicted maximum heart rate during exercise test), and its association with a high incidence of CAD and sudden cardiac death. Patients who take heart rate lowering medications like beta blockers and Digoxin were excluded from these observations. A poor heart rate response to exercise by itself does not mean that the test is invalid. Instead, it is an independent predictor of sudden death, and therefore it warrants further imaging or invasive investigations.

The mechanisms of chronotropic incompetence are unclear, except to say it reflects an incompetence of the autonomic modulations of heart function.

Sudden cardiac death syndrome, which in essence is death and resurrection—is a product and a miracle of modern medicine.

*If a free society cannot help the many who are poor,
it cannot save the few who are rich.*

**John F. Kennedy
(1917–1963)**

Chapter Seven

Some Questions...Some Thoughts

racticing as a cardiologist in Rochester, New York, for the last two decades, I have been posed with a variety of very interesting questions by my patients. It is intriguing to see how little our community knows when it comes to the most critical part of corpus humanus.

Missing and misinterpreting the early symptoms of a heart attack, thereby misdiagnosing and mistreating this disease is the greatest miss of all in medicine. "This will never happen to me"... "I can hack it with some antacids"... "It is only a chest cold"... "It looks like stomach upset"... "Some kind of a flu"... "I would rather have a drink"... "I didn't want to wake you up"... "I didn't want to bother anybody"...are some of the silent soliloquies of my patients in the early minutes of their symptoms while actually an acute heart attack was already in the making. Let me share with you some of these questions and my thoughts on them.

1. "My doctor did an EKG on me recently. Why didn't he detect the blockages?"

EKG is a good test to determine the rate and rhythm of the heart, evidence of thickness of the heart muscle, and the patency of the conducting system, and its abnormalities. It can also detect the location of previous heart attacks. In the beginning of a heart attack, it is of utmost use to identify changes, which has great therapeutic implications for administration of clot-busters. However, an EKG is not useful in detecting atherosclerotic blockages in coronary artery diseases with any confidence. In essence, EKG is not meant to detect atherosclerotic build-up or chronic subtotal blockages.

"I had a physical done...a little high cholesterol, but the EKG was fine, no heart problems, give me one more hamburger"...is not an unusual reaction amongst many of us. We have heard several stories of having had a normal physical with normal EKG and the person developing a heart attack or sustaining sudden death within hours or days.

EKG is a wonderful tool to identify whether a given coronary blockage is severely flow limiting particularly with exercise and unique in its ability to distinguish coronary anginal pain from atypical non-cardiac pains. The evaluation of an acute myocardial infarction is very closely monitored by serial EKGs. EKG is the quickest and most widely utilized bedside cardiac test of all kinds and times.

2. "My cholesterol is normal.
How did I get cholesterol build-up in my coronaries?"

Although people with hypercholesterolemia have a much higher incidence of coronary artery disease, hypercholesterolemia is not a must for atherosclerotic build-up in the coronary system. The term "cholesterol build-up" is an oversimplified version of the real fact. In fact, only 50% of hypercholesterolemic patients have symptomatic CAD, and in 50% of hypercholesterolemic patients there is no evidence of symptomatic CAD.

The inner lining of the coronary arteries (the endothelial cells) can become dysfunctional from many reasons including high blood pressure, high cholesterol, diabetes, cigarette smoking, family history of coronary artery disease, infections, etc. Via such dysfunctional endothelial cells, molecules of low-density lipoproteins (LDL) will gain access into the intima of the artery. Those intracellular LDL molecules are soon oxidized. The oxidized lipids are engulfed by monocytes in large quantities and transform them into foam cells. This initial reaction is followed by a cascade of interrelated reactions, resulting in vasoconstriction, migration and proliferation of smooth muscle cells. There will be further accumulation of lipids, monocytes, and macrophages, resulting in the formation of a plaque. This plaque is the common denominator in all forms of atherosclerotic vascular diseases irrespective of the site (coronaries or elsewhere). Sometimes these plaques are heavily impregnated with lipids, making it quite susceptible to rupture and hemorrhage. Such lipid-rich unstable plaques can cause any level of coronary instability including unstable angina, nontransmural myocardial infarction, transmural myocardial infarction, or sudden death. High cholesterol plays a very important role in the formation of cholesterol plaques in arteries, but hypercholesterolemia is not a must for atherosclerosis.

3. About cardiac catheterizations:

What is a cardiac catheterization?
What is coronary angiography?
What is a left heart catheterization?
What are the risks of an angiography?
Is there an age limit for coronary angiograms?

Cardiac catheterizations with coronary angiography are the ultimate diagnostic technique to determine whether a patient has CAD or not. Catheterization accurately delineates the location and degree of the blockages. We also get a very good idea about the morphology of the plaque; whether it is eccentric, concentric, calcified, soft, or burdened with thrombus.

The patients are prepared for the procedure with a medical history taking; physical examination; blood, EKG, and chest x-ray evaluations. They are asked to fast for approximately 12 hours prior to these procedures. Then, they are taken to a Cardiac Catheterization Laboratory. Under strict sterile precautions, a small catheter (a catheter is a preformed plastic tube of 2-3 mm in diameter) is inserted into the central aorta via the femoral or brachial artery. This entry of the catheter into the cardiovascular system is termed cardiac catheterization.

Under fluoroscopic control, this catheter is then advanced to the aortic root. The aortic root is the direct continuation of the left ventricle separated by the aortic valve. It is from the aortic root that the left and right coronary arteries take their origin. The two coronary arteries then divide into several branches, and eventually crown the heart—hence the name "coronary arteries." The left anterior

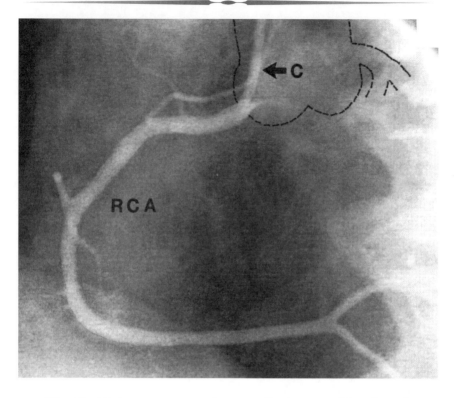

(**Fig. 9**)   Right coronary angiogram of a 48-year-old male with atypical complaints of chest pain.
C – catheter. **RCA** – right coronary artery.

Figure 9 is a normal right coronary angiogram. The right coronary artery supplies the atria, sinoatrial node, atrioventricular node, free wall of the right ventricle, the diaphragmatic portion of the left ventricle, and the lower intra-ventricular septum. Occlusion of the right coronary artery leads to a diaphragmatic myocardial infarction. Acute occlusion of the right coronary artery used to bear a mortality of at least 30% in the pre-thrombolytic and interventional era.

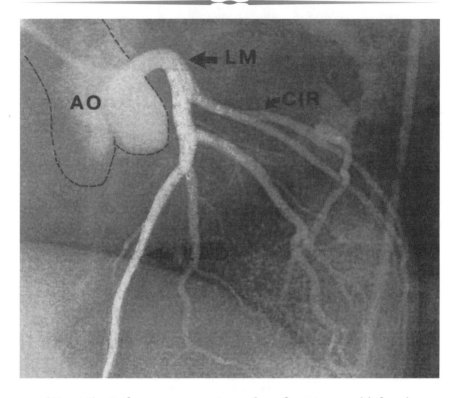

(**Fig. 10**) Left coronary angiography of a 90-year-old female showing diffuse coronary artery calcification without discrete stenosis.

AO – aorta. **CIR** – circumflex artery. **LAD** – left anterior descending artery. **LM** – left main coronary artery.

Figure 10 is a left coronary angiogram from a 90-year-old female. There was evidence of diffuse calcification on fluoroscopic examination. The angiogram did not show any evidence of discrete atherosclerosis. This is considered to be a "normal angiogram," although there is a very high likelihood of having some diffuse generalized atherosclerosis if you further examine this vessel from within by an intravascular ultrasound.

descending artery, circumflex artery (both coming from the left main coronary artery) and the right coronary artery are the three major coronary arteries. From these three major conduit vessels and their branches, several small vessels perforate into the myocardium to perfuse every segment of the heart muscle.

From the aortic root the catheter is then directed to the ostia of the coronary arteries. Iodine-containing contrast material is then directly injected into the vessel. Whereas the contrast material is occupying the lumen of the coronary arteries, discrete atherosclerotic plaques sticking into the lumen of the coronary artery will be identified as a filling defect—a lesion. When the contrast is flowing through the arteries, angiogram pictures are recorded by using an x-ray machine in a film or digital video format. This step is called coronary angiography.

The left main coronary artery and its branches supply 70-80% of the left ventricle—the main pumping chamber of the human heart.

A total occlusion of the left main coronary artery is fatal with a massive myocardial infarction unless the distal branches get a copious supply of collateral filling from the right coronary artery.

Sudden occlusion of the proximal LAD can also be fatal. A critical blockage on the proximal LAD used to be called a "widow maker." Now that we know CAD is an equal opportunity affliction, it must also be called a "widower maker" to be statistically and politically correct.

An occlusion of the circumflex can also be fatal. However, it is not just the amount of the myocardium in jeopardy that determines the mortality, but also the overall cardiac reserve ventricular function, vagal tone, and the propensity for ventricular fibrillation that finally determines the mortality of a given heart attack.

Cardiac catheterization is only a diagnostic procedure and not a treatment for coronary artery disease. The risk of mortality from this test is about 1 in 800 cases. Heart attack, stroke, aortic or coronary dissections, contrast reaction, and bleeding are the major complications.

There is no age limit for coronary angiograms in the United States. There are several countries in Europe and elsewhere where an upper age limit is set by health care rationing authorities, usually the government. We know that all humans are not created equal when it comes to the aging of the protoplasm. The physiological age of the person, the strength of the indication, and the desire of the patient must be the major factors in the decision-making process of performing an angiogram in an elderly person.

4. "My doctor did an exercise test on me recently and said it was normal. Now you did an angiogram and tell me that I have four blockages. Why is that?"

An exercise test is a good screening test to identify critical exercise-induced, flow-limiting blockages in the coronary system. If a patient has tight (more than 75%) blockage in one or more of the coronaries, an exercise test can induce some chest pain and/or EKG changes in about 25%-65% of the patients. A nuclear stress test or a stress echocardiography will improve the sensitivity of detecting coronary artery disease by 80%. In about 30% of the patients, even with critical blockages of the coronary arteries, an exercise test will not be very useful and may even be misleading by demonstrating a "normal" result. If a patient has one or more subcritical blockages, i.e., blockages less than 70%, an ETT may read entirely normal also.

A coronary angiogram is the one and only diagnostic test, which will absolutely identify the exact location and degree of coronary stenosis. In rare instances, one might even need an intravascular ultrasound examination for the most accurate evaluation of the degree, nature, and extent of coronary stenosis.

It is reasonable to say that an exercise test is **not** a test to identify build-up of cholesterol in the coronary system. **Even in those patients with very severe three-vessel coronary artery disease, a treadmill test could be read as normal.** This happens particularly when there is collateral circulation.

Case Study

A 58-year-old physically very active and totally asymptomatic

dentist had a minor EKG change (mild T wave inversion in the inferior leads) on the resting 12-lead EKG during annual physical examination. His life insurance policy was denied due to this change. He
had a perfectly normal treadmill exercise test, as well as stress
echocardiography with no evidence of exercise-induced chest pain,
anginal equivalent symptoms, or additional EKG changes. Still his
policy was denied. Subsequently, a nuclear exercise test showed multiple small reversible perfusion abnormalities in the myocardium.

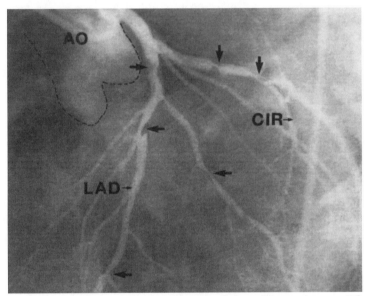

(**Fig. 11**) Coronary angiogram from this patient. The
angiogram showed normal systolic function of the left ventricle.
The right coronary artery was totally occluded with collaterals
from the left coronary artery. There were multiple 60-95%
stenoses on the left coronary system, as shown in the figure. He
underwent five-vessel CABG. He had some, if not, more T wave
changes on the EKG postoperatively.

Caveat – *New EKG changes, even if minor, must be evaluated thoroughly.*

5. How can we remove or correct those blockages in the coronary arteries?

CAD is a permanent and progressive disease. Once you have it, you just had it. Total removal of the atherosclerotic plaques by medications or devices will be the challenge of the present millennium. In rare instances, we are able to remove the critical portion of an atherosclerotic blockage by a device called **directional atherectomy**. In most such instances, the atheroma will grow back.

For thick and calcified blockages another device called **Rotablator** has been used to drill through the blockages using high speed, diamond-head, pear-shaped drilling balls with some success. None of these devices are capable of removing the atherosclerotic blockages completely or permanently. **Angio-Jet** is a relatively new device used to remove fresh blood clots from newly infarcted coronary arteries by using a flushing-suction technique. This is used as an adjunct for angioplasty.

Apart from risk factor modification, coronary revascularization techniques are the mainstay in the management of coronary artery disease.

Currently available revascularization techniques are listed below:

Percutaneous transluminal coronary angioplasty (PTCA).
Coronary stenting.
Coronary rotablation (Rotational atherectomy).
Directional atherectomy.
Intracoronary radiation therapy (Brachytherapy).
Transmyocardial laser recanalization (TMR).

hope of reducing casualties and saving lives. However, there are several other personal aspects of human behavior that cannot be regulated (e.g., smoking, alcohol, drugs, severe obesity), which could eventually translate into emergency room care draining millions of dollars from our health care treasure chest. The impact of gunshot wounds, stabbing, and other such violent activities on our health care system are just phenomenal.

> Just as we know that passive smoking (second-hand) can affect innocent, disciplined individuals in the community, ill health of a community member from any which reason will certainly affect you quite directly: by depleting the community reserves, hospital resources, higher premiums on health insurances, taxes, and the related whole nine-yards of it.

In essence, in a society where social security is an obligation, depletion of the community treasure chest must be your concern too. It is my belief that the community at large is receptive and responsive to public health initiatives if proper efforts are undertaken to educate them. The typical example of successful education is that of AIDS. The vast majority of the U.S. population now knows how AIDS is contracted, how it spreads, what its clinical manifestations are, how it is treated, and its overall prognosis.

> In essence, in a society where social security is an obligation, depletion of the community treasure chest must be your concern too.

Angiogenesis.

Eximer Laser coronary revascularization.

Above all, **coronary artery bypass graft surgery.**

Here, I would like to reemphasize that the fight against atherosclerosis is not just with angioplasty or the newer techniques; arresting the progression of atherosclerosis and even some regression has been demonstrated by coronary angiograms with meticulous lifestyle modification. Controlling cardiac risk factors particularly by cholesterol lowering medications, a very low fat diet, cessation of smoking, regular exercise, maintaining an ideal body weight, and stress management training are all found to be useful. Such aggressive lifestyle modifications are strongly recommended for patients with known CAD and those who are at high risk.

firmly believe that if all of the materia medica could be sent to the bottom of the sea, it would be all the better for mankind and all the worse for the fishes."

O.W. Holmes
(1841-1935)
Justice of the U.S. Supreme Court
Legal Historian and Philospher

6. <u>About angioplasties and stenting</u>:

How does a balloon work?

Do you keep the balloon in or take it out?

What happens to all the pieces of cholesterol that have been broken?

What is stenting?

How many vessels can be stented?

Do you take out the stent if it does not work?

What are rotorooters of the heart?

These are only a few of the long chain of questions that patients usually have with reference to this subject.

As we have discussed earlier on, coronary atherosclerosis leads to the formation of plaque. In general, there are two types of plaque formations with various levels of combinations. The first variety is discrete atherosclerosis, i.e., plaque formations that gradually invade the arterial lumen in an eccentric or concentric fashion. Such encroachment of the arterial lumen gradually reduces the lumen diameter to 50%, 70%, 90%, etc. Such discrete lesions are ideal for angioplasty. The second variety of plaque involvement is usually termed diffuse atherosclerosis, where many, if not almost all segments of the coronary arteries are involved in the atherosclerotic process, whereby the lumen is uniformly narrowed with few areas of discrete narrowing on top of the diffuse disease. Symptomatic discrete atherosclerotic lesions from around 60-99% of stenosis are ideal cases for balloon angioplasty.

Before angioplasty we obtain an angiogram in multiple views. The angiogram is then carefully reviewed to see how many blockages there are, the location, the degree of stenosis and morphology of these blockages.

Correlating the symptoms and the region of ischemia, a decision is made to open the appropriate blockages, employing angioplasty. In general, left main stenosis and multiple blockages involving all three major vessels, and diffuse blockages are not attempted for elective angioplasty.

Angioplasty is the endovascular remodeling of a clogged vessel by inflating a balloon against the blockage. Here, a special catheter very similar to a diagnostic angiography catheter is advanced to the ostia of the target coronary artery via the femoral artery or brachial artery. This tube has an internal diameter of about 3.0 mm. This catheter serves as a transport conduit for the necessary wires, balloons, stents, and other required hardware. It is through this same catheter that all necessary radiopaque contrast materials and medications are administered directly into the coronary arteries.

Once we have identified a target lesion to be opened up, a thin (14/1000 of an inch) flexible guidewire is slowly advanced through the artery, across the blockage, and the wire is parked in the whole extent of the vessel. Angioplasty balloons are available in various diameters (1.5 mm to 5.5 mm) and lengths (15 mm to 40 mm). An appropriate sized deflated balloon is then advanced to the blockage area by railing through the guidewire. The balloon is then inflated to break and compress the plaque against the wall. The balloon can be inflated anywhere from 3 to 24 atmospheres of pressure, and kept inflated in the arterial lumen from a few seconds to several minutes. When the balloon is inflated, the blood supply through that vessel is temporarily cut off. Then, the patient can have ischemic symptoms (chest pain, tightness, etc.). The balloon is then deflated and railed out through the existing guidewire. In balloon angioplasty, the cholesterol plaques are not taken out. They are ruptured and compressed against the wall. This area continues to heal by the body's own remodeling process, and finally covered by healthy endothelium from either end of the treatment area.

Balloon angioplasty has a 95% primary success rate, but the long-term patency is only 60%.

Coronary stenting

The primary failure of balloon angioplasty is due to a variety of factors including coronary spasm, elastic recoil of the vessel, and balloon-induced uncontrolled dissection of the arteries. This situation can be effectively handled by deployment of a stent into the balloon-treated area of the vessel.

A stent is a stainless steel slotted tube or coil meshwork made in different diameters and lengths. They are mounted on an angioplasty balloon in the deflated state. The stent is advanced via the guidewire railing system, and taken to the desired treatment area. The balloon is then inflated to expand the stent. The expanding power of the balloon deploys the stent into the internal layers of the artery. The balloon is then deflated and taken out. The expanded deployed stent remains in this vessel scaffolding it from within. The stent remains in the vessel forever. The guidewire is then finally pulled out. The primary success rate of coronary stenting is over 99%, and the long-term patency is about 80%. That is the reason why stenting is used in about 80% of all percutaneous coronary interventions. We can stent several vessels at the same sitting, or as a staged procedure in certain instances.

Case Studies:

Stenting of a right coronary artery lesion

A 55-year-old postmenopausal woman with strong family history of coronary artery disease presented with com-

plaints of left wrist pain and mild shortness of breath. She had
marked EKG changes and elevated cardiac enzymes consistent
with nontransmural myocardial infarction. Coronary
angiogram revealed a 95% stenosis of the mid right coronary
artery. This vessel was subjected for angioplasty and stenting.
I am using this case to demonstrate the stepwise procedure of
coronary stenting.

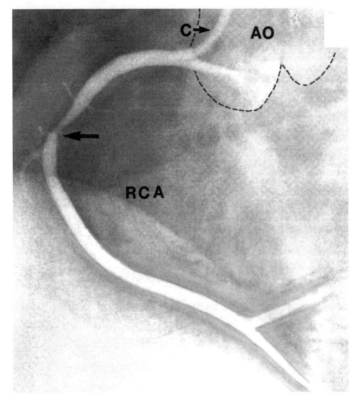

(Fig. 12A) RCA of a 55-year-old female—Selective right
coronary angiography showing a high-grade lesion of the mid
right coronary artery.
AR - aortic root. **C** - catheter. **RCA** - right coronary artery.
Arrow - 90% stenosis of the mid right coronary artery.

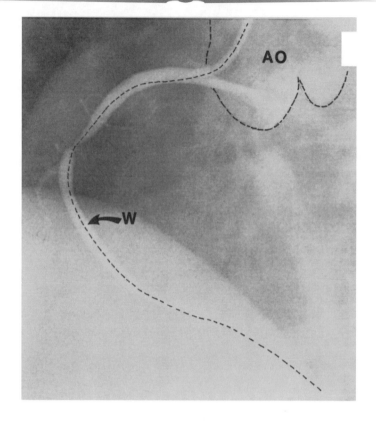

(**Fig. 12B**) Wiring.

W - wire.   A 0.014-inch diameter stainless steel guidewire is
passed through the blockage and parked all the way to the
distal portion of the right coronary artery. This wire will function as a "monorail" for the advancement of the balloon and
stent.

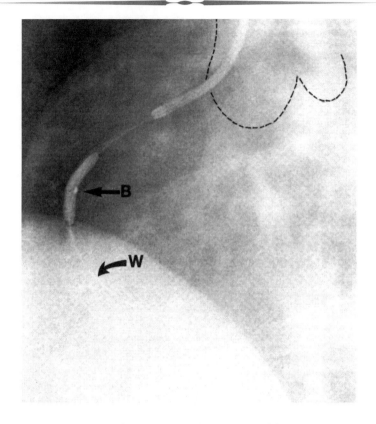

(Fig. 12C) Balloon angioplasty—Predilatation.

B – balloon. **W** – wire. A 20 mm long and 2.5 mm diameter (when inflated) balloon is placed at the site of the blockage and inflated up to 10 atmospheres. The balloon will split and compress the cholesterol plaque creating a space. In effect, this is balloon angioplasty. In this case we might call it predilatation, as we are planning to put a stent at this site.

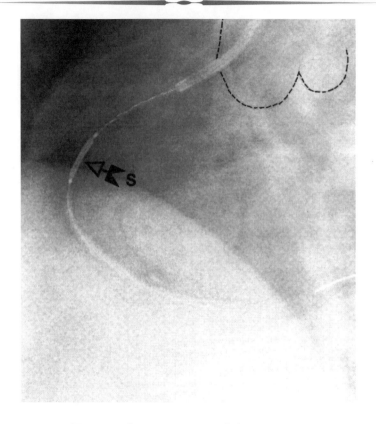

(**Fig. 12D**) Positioning of the stent.

A stent before deployment—A 3.5 mm diameter and 18 mm long stent mounted on a deflated balloon is placed at the original site of the blockage.

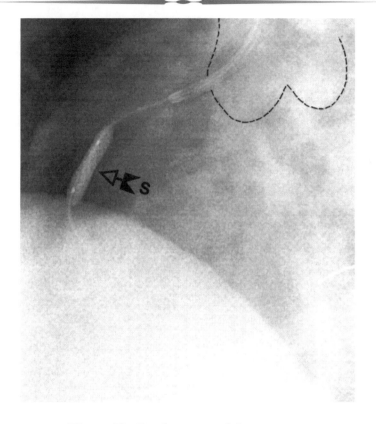

(Fig. 12E) Deployment of the stent.

S – stent. The stent-mounted balloon is then inflated up to 16 atmospheres for 30 seconds. The balloon is then deflated and taken out. The stent remains in the lumen of the artery scaffolding it from within.

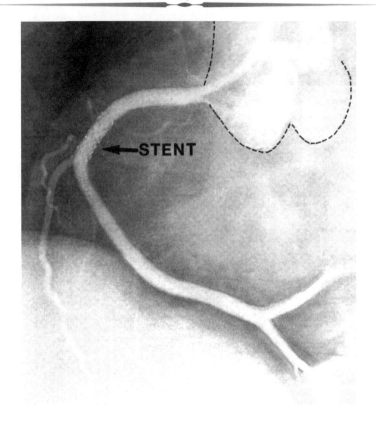

(**Fig. 12F**) The stented vessel.

The balloon and wire are now removed, and the stent is deployed in the target area. The angiogram shows a widely patent vessel with no evidence of any residual stenosis.

Complex Coronary Stenting

"Kissing stents"

A 60-year-old hypertensive female underwent a coronary angiogram as an investigation for her unstable angina. Figure 13A shows selective left coronary injection. The proximal portion of the left anterior descending artery is normal. This vessel then bifurcates into a diagonal branch. The white arrow in the figure shows 70%-80% complex lesions immediately before and after this bifurcation. The black arrow shows a plaque lesion on the circumflex vessel.

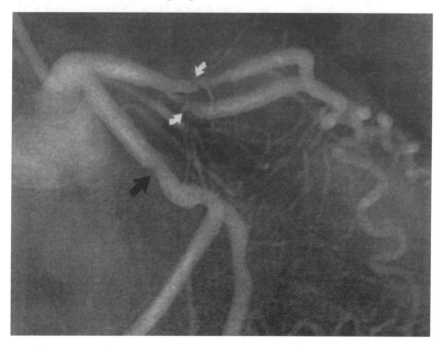

(**Fig. 13A**) White arrows—The left coronary angiogram of a 60-year-old woman having a complex stenosis involving the LAD and large diagonal branch.

The LAD-diagonal system was then subjected for angioplasty. The two vessels were then wired as described before. Then, two stents were simultaneously advanced into these blockages and placed in position. The two stents were then simultaneously inflated up to 14 atmospheres. Following deployment of the stent, the balloons were taken out. As shown in Figure 13B, following stenting, the two vessels are widely patent with no evidence of any residual stenosis. In this technique, two stents are placed side-by-side with their proximal ends touching and kissing each other—this technique is termed kissing stent.

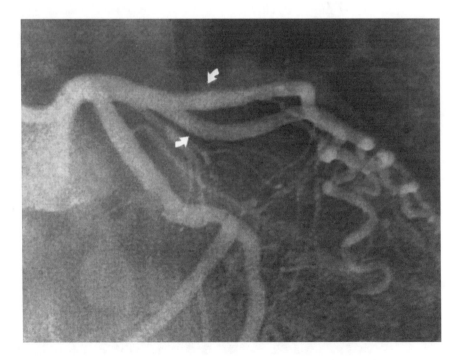

(**Fig. 13B**) The LAD-diagonal lesions are now fully reopened by simultaneous application of two stents in   the treatment area—kissing stents, as marked by the   white arrows.

Coronary Stenting Assisted by Intravascular Ultrasound

A 45-year-old man with history of hypertension and severe hypercholesterolemia was admitted to the hospital with acute coronary syndrome. Angiogram showed a 50% ulcerated lesion of the proximal LAD. He was medically treated, stabilized, and discharged. A week later he was readmitted with a nontransmural myocardial infarction. Angiogram again showed a 50% ulcerated lesion of the proximal LAD (Fig. 14A). He did not have any other blockages on the circumflex system or the right coronary artery. Intravascular

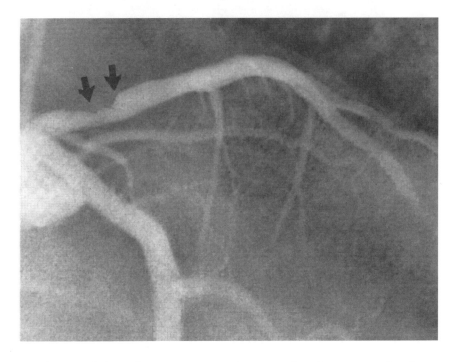

(**Fig. 14A**) Left coronary angiogram showing a proximal eccentric ulcerated 50% stenosis shown by the two black arrows.

ultrasound examination showed a 70% lipid-rich ulcerated lesion
(Fig. 14B—IVUS image). This lesion was stented with resolution of
the symptoms (Fig. 14C).

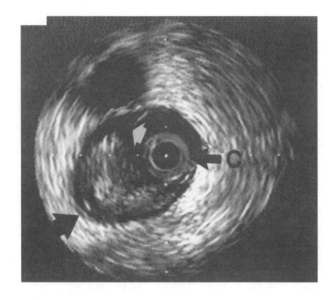

(**Fig. 14B**) Intravascular ultrasound showing plaque burden in
the lumen of the coronary artery.

C – catheter.   Black arrow – bulging of the coronary artery by
heavy plaque load.   White arrow – possible point of rupture
of a soft plaque.

Intravascular ultrasound is exceptionally useful to study the
morphology and extent of coronary lesions in selected cases. Here,
the angiogram showed only a 50% eccentric lesion, which is to be
treated medically as was done in this case. However, the angiogram
underestimated the severity of the lesion, and didn't give a clue as to
the instability of the plaque. The intravascular ultrasound showed

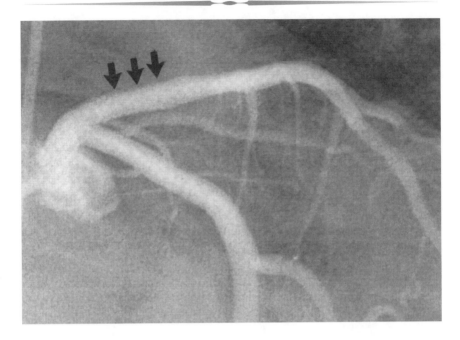

(**Fig. 14C**) Following stenting, the left anterior descending artery is widely patent as shown by the three black arrows.

that the plaque burden has already remodeled the coronary artery making the cross-sectional view of oval shape rather than circular, and that the plaque is soft, lipid-rich, and without calcium.

Moreover, we can see the point of plaque rupture at the 11 o'clock position—small white arrow. It was this rupture that resulted in acute coronary syndrome in this patient.

Case Study

Primary Angioplasty / Stenting

A 55-year-old diabetic and hypertensive female with morbid obesity developed severe shortness of breath, chest tightness, diaphoresis, and then fainted. Paramedics arrived within six minutes of a 911 call. The patient was in full cardiac arrest with ventricular fibrillation. She received CPR and was electrically cardioverted 11 times. The patient was then intu-

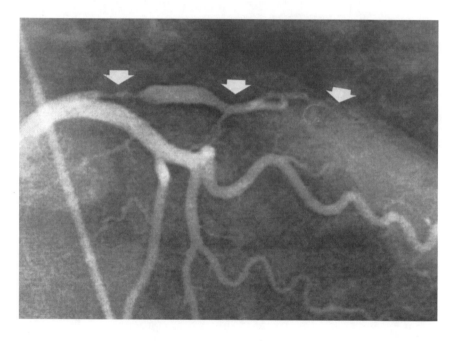

(**Fig. 15A**) Selective left coronary angiogram shows subtotal occlusion of a large left anterior descending coronary artery, as shown by the white arrows.

bated, medically stabilized in the best possible way, and was taken to the Cath Lab at Rochester General Hospital for an emergency angioplasty. She had a totally occluded right coronary artery. The LAD was the target lesion of the present myocardial infarction. This vessel was totally occluded as shown in Figure 15A (white arrows). This blockage was opened and stented establishing excellent antegrade flow as in Figure 15B. This patient walked out of the hospital on the fourth day in stable condition. This patient was critically ill with rapid deterioration into ventricular fibrillation and cardiac arrest.

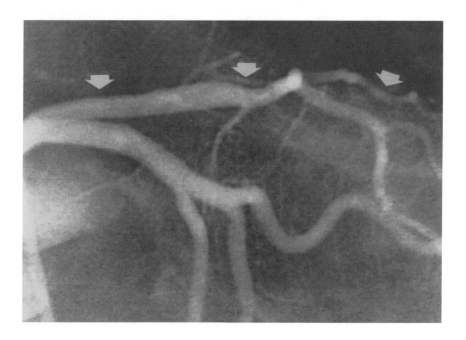

(**Fig. 15B**) Following coronary stenting, the LAD is widely patent with all its branches as shown by the white arrows.

Such patients are not candidates for thrombolytic therapy. They are best treated by medical stabilization and emergency angioplasty with or without stenting. This procedure of directly opening up a clogged vessel in a patient without giving thrombolytic therapy is called primary angioplasty or primary stenting if a stent is used.

In addition to balloon angioplasty and stenting, there are several other adjuncts we use in an interventional lab to offer patients the most optimal care.

Directional atherectomy is a cutting device occasionally used to take out pieces of athcrosclerotic plaques from the coronary arteries.

Rotational atherectomy (Rotablation device) is a diamondhead, pear-shaped, metallic ball called a bur that is advanced to the coronary artery by a guidewire railing system. The bur is then drilled through the plaque at a speed of 150,000–180,000 rotations per minute. The drilling will make the plaque into extremely small particles of 1 micron or less. These particles will flow down distally, and eventually be engulfed by the other cells and destroyed (phagocytosis).

Another important device that we use in the lab is an **intracoronary ultrasound device**. A small transducer of 1.5 mm in size is advanced through the coronary artery via a guidewire railing system. The piezoelectric crystals in the transducer are then activated to obtain ultrasound images of the artery. This device is extremely useful in several instances where we want to learn more about a given lesion before and after angioplasty or stenting.

7. <u>What is cath-plasty?</u>

Cardiac catheterization is only a diagnostic technique, whereas angioplasty (including stenting, Rotablation, etc.) is a definitive treatment to open up partially or completely clogged vessels. Cardiac catheterization is an invasive procedure which demands a lot of preparation including blood work, chest x-ray, fasting for over 12-hours, pre-medications, and insertion of venous lines for fluids and medications, and finally several catheters into the central aortic circulation for angiography.

In many Cath Labs, coronary angiograms are done on one day, and coronary interventions at a later date in the same hospital or another hospital. There are many reasons to do so:

a. The Cath Labs do not have interventional services.
b. The physician is not trained in interventional procedures.
c. The physician thinks it is better to delay the procedure so that the angiograms can be better studied.
d. Physician and hospital reimbursement is better with dual procedures, as they do two procedures on two different days.
e. Some low volume Interventional Cath Labs may not have enough rooms or may not have sufficient facilities for a diagnostic procedure to proceed into an interventional procedure, which will demand a lot more time and personnel.

It makes all the more sense, better patient safety and convenience, when angiograms and angioplasties are done.

Cardiac catheterization is never a benign procedure. It is attended by complications of mortality (1 in 800 patients), stroke (1 in 500 patients), heart attack (1 in 500 patients), catheter-induced coronary dissection (1 in 1,000 patients), groin complications of bleeding requiring blood transfusion, and compromise of the femoral or brachial artery circulation requiring surgery, and occasional major contrast reactions. In addition, there are also chances of infection and deterioration of kidney function in some cases.

Cath-Plasty

It is the way to go for all future interventions. Less preparation time. Less hospital time. Single invasion. One hospital fee. One physician fee. Better patient satisfaction. Less combined complications. Saving dollars.

Some of these complications, particularly coronary artery dissection and acute occlusions are better handled in an Interventional Lab, which has the backup of an Angioplasty Service and Cardiothoracic Surgical Team. Therefore, it makes all the more sense, better patient safety and convenience, when angiograms and angioplasties are done in the same lab in the same sitting. By doing so, the patient needs to be prepared and pre-medicated only once, and moreover the arterial system to be invaded only once. This combined procedure of angiogram and angioplasty in the same sitting is commonly called cath-plasty.

In addition to better patient convenience, safety, less lab and hospital time, a less incidence of combined morbidity and mortality is also noted with cath-plasty. Cath-plasty also saves about $4000.00 to $5,000.00 per patient rather than when angiogram and angioplasty are done as separate procedures.

When CAD patients are properly selected and processed for coronary angiography, 40-50% of them are candidates for percutaneous interventions of angioplasty or stenting, about 30% of them are candidates for bypass graft surgery, and the remaining are for medical management.

Combining angiogram and angioplasty in the same sitting (cath-plasty) is the fastest growing segment of interventional work in any major cath lab in the United States, like Rochester General Hospital in New York.

I have been practicing this discipline of combining angiograms (diagnostic tests) and angioplasties (a treatment procedure) in the same sitting for the last decade to the best of satisfaction and convenience to my patients, families, and referring physicians.

8. About coronary bypass graft surgery

Does the surgeon remove my blockages?
Is my artery replaced by the vein graft?
How many grafts can be placed?
How long is the operation good for?
What is the benefit of using the internal mammary artery
    for a bypass graft?

The coronary arteries are the first set of blood vessels, originating from the root of the aorta, to exclusively perfuse the heart muscles with blood. These arteries with their major branches are placed on the exterior of the heart like a crown—hence the name coronary arteries. The major conduit vessels have numerous branches perforating into the heart muscle, supplying blood all the way to the interior of the heart muscle.

Atherosclerotic blockages can be present anywhere in the system, in small, medium, or large vessels, as identified by coronary angiography. By carefully studying an angiogram, a surgeon can determine the arteries that can be bypass grafted. The surgeon does not remove any of the blockages nor replace any of the arteries. The surgeon procures a piece of saphenous vein 6-8 inches in length from the patient's leg. One end of this vein graft is then anastamosed to the aorta, and the other end to the coronary artery distal to the blockage. Through this newly constructed route, blood will freely flow to the coronary artery bypassing the blockage; hence the name aortocoronary saphenous vein bypass graft, as shown in Fig. 16A.

There is no absolute limit for the number of blockages that can be bypass grafted. I knew one patient who had nine bypass

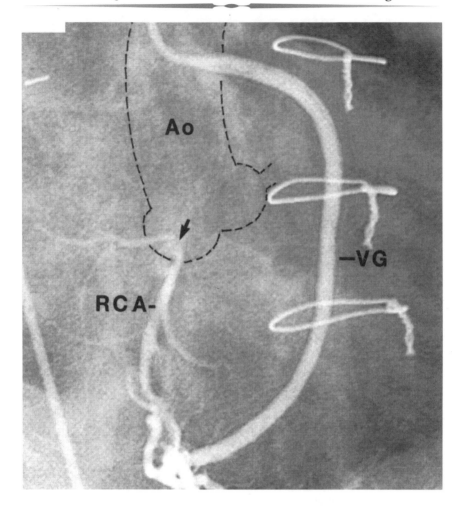

(**Fig. 16A**) Anatomy of a bypass graft.
Aortocoronary saphenous vein bypass graft.

AO – aorta overdrawn into the angiogram.   **RCA** – right coronary artery.   **VG** – vein graft.   Black arrow – the ostia of the right coronary artery.

grafts—the maximum I have seen. There are three major vessels in the coronary system (the left anterior descending artery, the circumflex artery, and the right coronary artery) that most often are subjected to bypass grafting. Several branches of these vessels, such as diagonals, marginals, posterior descending, etc., are also often grafted. However, a surgeon cannot graft all the blockages in some patients due to diffuse disease, and the small caliber or heavy calcification of the vessels. Generally, a coronary artery less than 1 mm in diameter is almost impossible to be grafted. In essence, even after multivessel bypass grafting, there could be several more small vessels with blockages ungrafted due to technical reasons. That is the reason why some patients, even after bypass graft surgery, could have residual symptoms or demonstrable ischemia.

Coronary bypass using the internal mammary artery

The **left internal mammary artery (LIMA)** originates from the proximal left subclavian artery and is meant to supply the left anterior chest wall. This arterial supply is not an absolute must for the chest wall. Therefore, this artery can be liberated from the chest wall, and can be directly grafted to the left anterior artery of the heart, thereby establishing a **direct arterial conduit** to the coronary artery. This graft lasts for several decades and is somewhat immune to atherosclerosis. Nowadays, the surgeons make every effort to put a LIMA graft in favor of its longevity (Fig. 16B).

Vein grafts have a tendency to undergo dilatation, thrombosis, intimal hyperplasia, degeneration, atherosclerosis, and occlusion in a somewhat predictable way. The leg veins are very thin-walled conduits, meant to carry blood to the heart under very low pressure of 3-5 mmHg. When these tubes are placed into high-pressured arterial systems (120-222 mmHg or more, depending on the blood pressure of the patient), they undergo the above-mentioned changes very quickly.

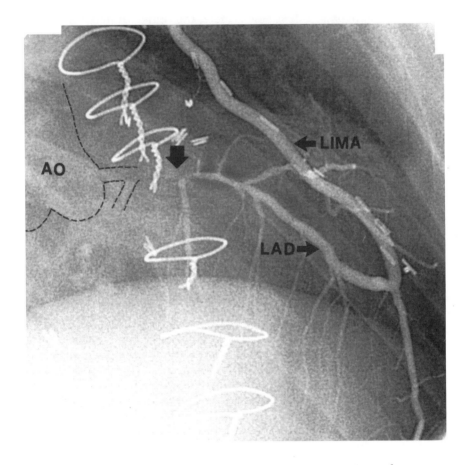

(**Fig. 16B**) Internal mammary artery anastamosis to the left anterior descending artery.

AO – aorta. **LAD** – left anterior descending artery. **LIMA** – left internal mammary artery. Black arrow – total blockages of the proximal LAD.

<u>Case Studies</u>

The figure shows selective vein graft injection of a 70-year-old female. Angiogram performed three years after the initial bypass graft surgery. Here, the right coronary artery is diffusely diseased in its proximal and mid portions. The ostium has a 95% stenosis. A piece of vein is harvested from the leg. One end of the vein is anastamosed to the aorta and the other end to the distal right coronary artery. This graft has now bypassed the lesion of the right coronary artery, and reaches blood to the distal portions of the right coronary artery; hence the term aortocoronary saphenous vein bypass graft surgery.

Figure 16B is an angiogram of a 78-year-old man with history of hypertension, hypercholesterolemia, and prior history of cigarette smoking. He had multivessel bypass graft surgery in 1989 with insertion of LIMA to the LAD, and aortocoronary saphenous vein bypass graft to the first marginal, second marginal, and the right coronary artery.

The angiogram done in August 2000 showed that all vein grafts are diffusely diseased or occluded. However, the LIMA was widely patent perfusing the LAD system. The LIMA looks pristine with no evidence of stenosis or atherosclerosis. This patient is dependent on this single graft.

9. <u>How long does CABG last</u>?

We have over thirty years of experience with coronary artery bypass graft surgery since its introduction in 1967. Bypassing a coronary blockage by insertion of a graft (bypass graft operation) is accomplished by two types of conduits: the arteries or the veins. An arterial conduit employing the internal mammary artery lasts the longest. At the end of 10 years, over 90% of the LIMA grafts are patent. In fact, we have seen many patients with an internal mammary graft surviving well over a quarter of a century, with no evidence of atherosclerotic build-up.

On the contrary, the vein graft conduits do degenerate faster with atherosclerotic changes, resulting in thrombosis and occlusion. In general, at the end of the first year after the operation 10-15% of the vein grafts are occluded; at the end of fifth year 40% of the vein grafts are occluded; however, by the tenth year nearly 75% of the vein grafts are occluded. Approximately 50% of the people will need a second revascularization process, either by bypass graft surgery or by angioplasty by the tenth postoperative year.

Arterial conduits last longer because they are designed to handle high-pressure arterial circulation, whereas veins are genetically meant to carry venous blood, which has very low luminal pressure. These thin-walled vein grafts when interposed in a relatively high-pressured arterial circulation, such as in coronary artery bypass graft surgery, undergo degenerative changes, dilatation, thrombosis, intimal hyperplasia, and atherosclerosis. That is the reason why these days more arterial conduits are being used by cardiac surgeons for coronary artery bypass graft surgery. The commonly used arterial conduits are the internal mammary arteries, radial arteries, and gastroepiploic arteries.

Case Studies

The following two case studies demonstrate the differentials in the degree of dilatation and degeneration between a vein graft and an arterial graft used for aortocoronary bypass graft surgery.

This 54-year-old man with history of cigarette smoking, hypertension, hypercholesterolemia, and overweight had three- vessel CABG in February 2000 for unstable angina. LIMA was inserted to the LAD, saphenous vein graft to the right coronary artery, and saphenous vein graft to the circumflex-marginal in sequence. The patient was readmitted with acute coronary syndrome five months after the surgery. The angiogram (Fig. 17A) now shows the saphenous vein graft to the right coronary artery is totally occluded, LIMA to the LAD is widely patent, saphenous vein graft to the circumflex-marginal system is patent. However, the vein graft as shown in the figure is quite markedly dilated with sluggish flow.

The saphenous vein with its very thin wall is not meant to function as an arterial conduit with very high intraluminal pressure (210/120 mmHg, as in this case). The vein graft then undergoes dilatation, tortuosity, thrombosis, intimal hyperplasia, atherosclerosis, and finally occlusion. When a vein graft is harvested from its natural habitat, the manipulation and disruption of its own native blood supply are all responsible cofactors. However, in my observation, patients harboring high blood pressure degenerate their vein grafts much quicker.

Even in patients with the worst cardiac risk factors, atherosclerosis in the venous system (not harvested) producing blockages is
virtually unheard of.   However, when they are removed and grafted

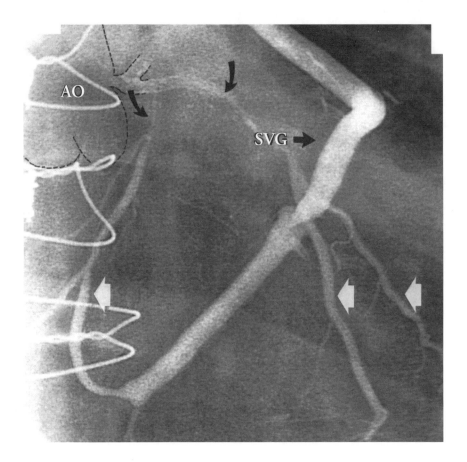

(**Fig.** 17A) Aortocoronary bypass vein graft to the marginal
system
AO – aorta.   **SVG** – saphenous vein graft.   Black bent arrows –
proximal occlusion of the circumflex marginal system.   White
arrows – the marginal branches of the circumflex artery.

into a high-pressure system, they undergo quite significant changes, as we had discussed earlier. Whereas all other cardiac risk factors remain the same, pretty much the only difference this harvested vein graft experiences is the high intraluminal pressure because of its interposition in the arterial system. In my opinion, hypertension is the worst atherosclerotic risk factor for vein grafts. (This is not confirmed or disputed by any studies.)

In my practice, I have seen only two cases (both postmortem) where some significant atherosclerosis of 40-50% was observed in the pulmonary arteries. Pulmonary arteries, in fact, are extensions of the body's venous system carrying impure blood from the heart to the lungs for purification. The pulmonary arterial wall is thicker than the systemic veins, but much thinner than similar sized systemic arteries. Their luminal pressure is also somewhat in between (25-35 mmHg) venous and arterial pressures. The two cases I mentioned had severe pulmonary hypertension of 70-80 mmHg. This rise in pressure, I believe, is the sole reason for the development of atherosclerotic blockages in pulmonary arteries in these patients.

I have given great emphasis to keep the blood pressure to the bare bottom level of 120 mmHg in everybody, particularly those after a bypass graft surgery. Remember, by the tenth postoperative year, well over 75% of the vein grafts will be either totally occluded or significantly diseased. Using aspirin from the second postoperative day onwards has shown significant benefit in reducing vein graft occlusions.

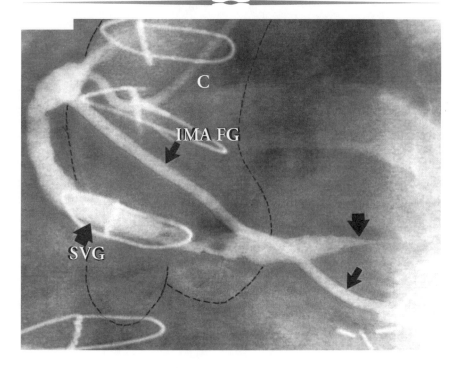

(**Fig. 17B**) Aortocoronary bypass graft. The saphenous vein graft is bypassed to the circumflex-marginal system. The internal mammary is used as a free graft from the aortic root to the mid LAD.

IMAFG – internal mammary artery free graft. **SVG** – saphenous vein graft. Thick arrows – 99% stenosis of the saphenous vein. Thin arrow – widely patent internal mammary artery used as a free graft. **C** - Catheter.

This angiogram is from a 68-year-old patient weighing 258 pounds with history of hypertension, hypercholesterolemia, family history of coronary artery disease, and extensive peripheral vascular disease who had multivessel bypass graft surgery in 1995. His CABG consisted of a saphenous vein graft to the circumflex-marginal, saphenous vein graft to the distal right coronary artery, and internal mammary artery used as a free graft to the LAD. In the usual circumstances, the internal mammary artery is directly anastamosed to the coronary artery, such that the blood freely flows from the brachial artery to the coronary artery. In this case, the internal mammary artery is used as an aortocoronary conduit because this patient had atherosclerotic disease in the left proximal subclavian artery.

At the time of this study in August 2000, the patient already had sustained a diaphragmatic myocardial infarction and had developed congestive heart failure with an ejection fraction of 45%. The saphenous vein graft to the right coronary artery was totally occluded. The saphenous vein graft to the circumflex-marginal system was dilated, tortuous, atherosclerotic, and critically stenosed with significant intraluminal load of thrombus.

In essence, the two venous conduits are totally dysfunctional. However, the arterial conduit (IMAFG) looked pristine, as a normal smooth conduit without any of the degenerative changes that happened to the venous system. Dr. David Cheeran, a senior cardiothoracic surgeon at Rochester General Hospital had the following comments on the subject. "Of course, internal mammary artery is the best conduit when it is directly anastamosed to the coronary artery. IMA or any other arterial conduits such as a the radial artery, when used as a free graft, fares much better than the saphenous vein grafts, but not as good as direct anastamosis of the internal mammary artery. The saphenous veins in some, particularly obese patients, are very large at the time of harvest, such vein grafts may degenerate much quicker particularly in a hypertensive."

Although the saphenous vein grafts degenerate in a predictable fashion, it certainly is not a universal phenomenon. I have seen several vein grafts, fifteen or twenty years after the bypass graft, working quite well with no evidence of degenerative changes. It is my feeling that CABG using medium-sized healthy vein grafts in subjects without hypertension or diabetes, and who do not smoke, last longer than the rest.

edicine is a collection of uncertain prescriptions, the result of which taken collectively are more fatal than useful to mankind.

Napoleon Bonaparte
(1769-1821)

10. Can infection produce heart attacks?

Much has been talked about the role of infection in the etiology of CAD and acute myocardial infarction, more so in the newspapers and television media rather than in medical literature.

Although we know that CAD is much more prevalent in high-risk groups, it will not account for about 50% of the patient population who have no conventional cardiac risk factors. Our great emphasis on cholesterol reduction with the use of statins did not start until the early 1990s. Aggressive efforts in blood pressure reduction did not start until the late 1970s. Smoking cessation, at the very best, is partially successful only since the late 1980s. Of course, the prevalence of obesity is certainly on the rise since we have been keeping track of it.

However, it is quite interesting to see that in the United States the coronary epidemic that was rampant in the 1950s peaked out in 1963, and ever since has shown a steady decline. This raises some logical questions: What exactly is the major force in this spectacular decline in CAD incidence? Is it due to the liberal and widespread use of antibiotics for so many common conditions? Is there a link between infection and CAD? Is the rise and fall of CAD in the 1950s and early 1960s related to prolonged infectious conditions not properly accounted for?

Amongst a few infectious agents investigated, the bacteria Chlamydia pneumoniae, which is responsible for as much as 10% of the community-acquired pneumonia is linked to atherosclerosis and myocardial infarction. Several studies have proved that men with AMI have increased seropositivity for Chlamydia pneumoniae than the control group. This bug has been isolated from 50-79% of the atherectomy specimens in some studies. There have even been some studies that show reduced incidence of myocardial infarction and angina in subjects treated with antibiotics (Azithromycin) when compared to the control group. However, the antibiotics used also

> It is quite interesting to see that in the United States the coronary epidemic that was rampant in the 1950s peaked out in 1963, and ever since has shown a steady decline.

have some anti-inflammatory effect, and therefore the full credit cannot be attributed to the bactericidal properties.

Inflammation and C-reactive protein

There is a growing body of information that suggests atherosclerosis is an inflammatory disease, infectious or not. Therefore, identifying markers of inflammation in the serum can predict acute coronary syndromes. C-reactive protein is a serum marker of inflammation somewhat nonspecific seen in various types of arthritis, infections, and inflammation of the atherosclerotic plaques.

High sensitivity C-reactive proteins and elevated fibrinogen levels have a predictive value for future coronary events and death. In many high-risk patients such as diabetics and smokers, there exists a chronic low-grade inflammation resulting in sustained elevation of C-reactive protein and fibrinogen. However, it is safe to assume that with a positive high sensitivity C-reactive protein, the atherosclerotic plaque may be unstable due to inflammation.

At this point we do not know what to do with this data. Until further convincing data is at hand, there is no specific recommendation to treat all patients with angina or MI with an antibiotic.

From exertion comes wisdom and purity, from sloth ignorance and sensuality.

Henry David Thoreau
(1817-1862)

11. Can exercise produce heart attacks?

Can exercise induce heart attacks?
Is exercise dangerous in survivors of heart attacks?
How much exercise could a heart attack patient do?
These are some of the concerns and questions I hear with
respect to exercise and heart attacks.

About 50% of all acute MIs are "triggered" by activities or adverse situations, which are commonly called "acute risk factors."

Vigorous physical activity in a deconditioned patient accounts for about 10-20% of acute myocardial infarctions as a trigger factor. In addition, severe emotional stress, earthquakes, and acute exposure to cold weather are well-recognized trigger factors. It is noted that the early morning hours of the first working day of the week (Monday) also has a trigger effect with increased incidence of acute myocardial infarctions.

While it is well known from epidemiological studies that habitual physical activity that conditions the cardiovascular system can reduce the incidence of myocardial infarction and sudden cardiac death in the general population, it might appear paradoxical when I say that vigorous physical activity, particularly in adverse conditions, can actually increase the incidence of myocardial infarction and sudden cardiac death. Whereas acute myocardial infarctions happen during or immediately after vigorous physical activity, strenuous physical activity becomes one of the most important triggers of an acute myocardial infarction.

An asymptomatic diabetic smoker with sedentary habits, who has hyperlipidemia and evidence of heart failure, constitutes the parameters of a person who has a high potential to develop exercise-induced myocardial infarctions. It is felt that rupture of a lipid-rich coronary plaque is responsible for the sudden deterioration into myocardial infarction and sudden cardiac death in this subset of patients. Angiography and postmortem studies have shown that these patients were more likely to have single-vessel coronary artery disease rather than three-vessel disease, and that they had more chance of having a blood clot in the infarct-related vessel.

> An asymptomatic diabetic smoker with sedentary habits, who has hyperlipidemia and evidence of heart failure, constitutes the parameters of a person who has a high potential to develop exercise-induced MIs.

Normally exercise increases the diameter of the coronary arteries, and the blood flow increases multifold. In addition, the bodies' own built-in clot-lysing factors are also activated. However, in a sedentary smoker, exercise can lead to real constriction of the vessels (exercise-induced coronary spasm), and can even trigger clot formation by stimulating the platelets (exercise-induced platelet aggregation). Moreover, the rapid rise in heart rate and blood pressure associated with strenuous exercise can exponentially increase the shearing forces in the coronary system creating a cleft in the cholesterol plaque leading to erosion, rupture, thrombosis, and occlusion of the artery resulting in an acute myocardial infarction.

In general, we can give some recommendations to individuals who are predisposed to exercise-induced acute myocardial infarction:

1. Individuals with high risk for myocardial infarction and sudden death must be aware of such situations and avoid unaccustomed vigorous exercise.

2. Modify cardiac risk factors as described above.

3. Must have a formal treadmill exercise test (TET) by a cardiologist before undertaking graded levels of exercise. The patient must follow some guidelines pertaining to the duration of exercise and the maximum pulse rate during exercise. These guidelines can be generated from a formal TET.

Case History

I have witnessed the tragic story of a 39-year-old gentleman weighing 340 pounds, a diabetic, heavy smoker with hyperlipidemia, who came to a cardiologist's office for the first treadmill exercise test. He ran for 3 minutes with a heart rate of 158 and blood pressure of 220/100. During the late recovery phase he had minor EKG changes of about 1.0 mm of ST depression with moderate shortness of breath. The young cardiologist prescribed aspirin, calcium channel blockers, and nitrates, and sent him home. On the way to the parking lot, the patient collapsed with a cardiac arrest. CPR was initiated within a few seconds. He was taken to the ED, which was very close by. With the full support of the ACLS team, resuscitation was attempted, but finally unsuccessful. Postmortem examination revealed severe three-vessel coronary artery disease, with almost a fully occluded circumflex artery with a fresh clot in it. It is concluded that this patient had a plaque rupture at the time of exercise leading to AMI and death. He did not have chest pain most likely due to diabetes.

Caveat

After having noted minor EKG changes late in the recovery phase of the exercise, it would have been ideal to delay the final EKG for another thirty minutes before the patient left the office.

It is very difficult to make predictions, particularly when it refers to the future.

Dan Quayle

12. <u>Could you predict sudden cardiac arrest?</u>

Foretelling the future of a disease process in a patient is one of the foremost duties of a physician. However, when it comes to the issue of coronary artery disease and sudden cardiac death, it is extremely difficult to predict the possibility of sudden cardiac death with any level of accuracy. As we have discussed before, of the half a million lives lost each year from coronary artery disease, approximately 250,000 of them did not have any symptoms or evidence of coronary artery disease or cardiovascular events in the past. In general, people who have a constellation of conventional as well as novel cardiac risk factors have a much higher incidence of coronary artery disease, and therefore SCD. In addition, a high resting heart rate of more than 84 beats per minute, diminished pumping function of the heart, a depressed heart rate variability, a high frequency of premature ventricular complex rates, left ventricular hypertrophy (LVH) on 12-lead EKG, nonspecific T wave inversions on the resting EKG, abnormal signal-average EKGs with late potentials, presence of significant plaque load on the carotid artery by ultrasound examination, ankle brachial index of less than 0.7, the presence of coronary calcification on ultrafast scanning, and high levels of fibrinogen and C-reactive proteins are all markers for coronary artery disease that are helpful to predict future coronary events in a subject.

If a person already has sustained a myocardial infarction it is easier to predict subsequent coronary events by identifying the following predictors:

1. <u>Ventricular fibrillation and ventricular tachycardia.</u> Patients with acute myocardial infarction developing VT or VF in the convalescent phase are at very high

risk to develop sudden cardiac death. Thirty-three percent of these patients sustain sudden cardiac arrest per year in the succeeding years.

2. <u>Out of hospital cardiac arrest</u>. If a patient is a survivor of an out of hospital cardiac arrest, he or she has about a 27% chance of developing a sudden cardiac death per year of survival; a situation considered to be very high risk.

3. <u>Poor pumping function and ventricular irritability</u>. Survivors of acute myocardial infarction with poor pumping function of the heart (ejection fraction 30% or below), and significant ventricular irritability (more than 10 premature ventricular beats per hour detected by an ambulatory Holter monitor evaluation) have a combined 50% risk of mortality for the next three years. However, survivors of acute myocardial infarction with good pumping function and having no ventricular irritability are also at a relatively high risk for sudden cardiac arrest—a cumulative 5% for the succeeding three years. It is important to note that this subset constitutes a very large number of patients, and therefore the total life loss is very high in this group.

4. <u>Poor heart rate variability</u>. In normal subjects, the beat-to-beat heart rhythm shows minor variations based on an intact sympathovagal system. This variability is quite marked with each respiration, physical activity, ischemia, and circadian rhythm. The heart's rhythm, contractility, and electrical stability are main-

tained by a balanced rich supply of sympathetic and parasympathetic fibers from the nervous system. The vagal reflex (parasympathetic activity mediated through the tenth cranial nerve) has a protective effect on ventricular irritability and fibrillation. Blunted heart rate variability is a manifestation of poor vagal tone. In survivors of an acute myocardial infarction, poor heart rate variability is associated with a high incidence of sudden cardiac death. There is a subset of patients who have distinctly poor heart rate variability response (HRV) in the early morning hours of the circadian rhythm, which correlates with the observation of an increased incidence of acute myocardial infarction and sudden cardiac arrest in the early morning hours. Now, we have the capabilities to assess poor heart rate variability with present day Holter monitors.

5. Late potentials and repetitive ventricular forms. In addition to poor heart rate variability, the presence of late potentials in a signal-average EKG, and repetitive ventricular forms are also independent markers of sudden cardiac arrest in survivors of acute myocardial infarction. However, the prognostic value is blunted by their poor specificity.

Can we predict a sudden cardiac arrest in the asymptomatic individual?

Of the 300,000 sudden cardiac deaths in the United States, the vast majority of them never experienced a cardiac event. **The overall incidence** of sudden cardiac death in the population at large is 0.1% to 0.2%, approximately one victim per year per 1,000 population. For the **high cardiac risk factor groups** (i.e., individuals with high blood pressure, diabetes, hypercholesterolemia, smoking, family history, etc.), who never sustained a cardiac event, the incidence of sudden cardiac death is about 16 per 1,000 population (1.6% per year). But the travesty of the situation is that a large section of the population is harboring high blood pressure, diabetes, and hypercholesterolemia even without being detected. They continue to smoke with a sense of impunity and never exercise, and thereafter will not know whether they have any exercise-induced symptoms at all.

As of now, we neither have a skin test to detect CAD nor a vaccine to prevent the disease. The risk factors must be screened and rectified. The individual's responsibility must be addressed and accepted.

In general, I can say that the following situations are predictors of coronary artery disease and consequently sudden cardiac arrest with very wide ranges of sensitivity and specificity.

1. Strong family history of premature coronary artery disease.
2. Smoking.
3. Diabetes.
4. High blood pressure.

5. Hyperlipidemic syndrome.
6. Obesity.
7. Postmenopausal state.
8. Sedentary habits.
9. Type A personality.
10. High dietary salt intake.
11. Novel cardiac risk factors. (See Chapter 3)
12. Left ventricular hypertrophy.
13. Abnormal resting heart rate (above 84 beats/min).
14. Carotid and peripheral vascular disease.
15. Reduced ankle brachial blood pressure index.
16. Poor chronotropic response with an exercise test.
17. Inappropriate heart rate recovery immediately after an exercise test (i.e., less than 12-beat reduction of the pulse rate in one minute after the peak exercise).
18. Elevated C-reactive protein and fibrinogen levels.

Above all, the individual's awareness of coronary artery disease and its implications deserve maximum attention.

Heart attacks without chest pain

About 33% of all heart attacks are without any chest pain. The incidence is very high if you are: an older person, a female, a diabetic, and have a history of congestive heart failure.

The impact: These patients reach the hospital late; more chance of misdiagnosis; less thrombolytic therapy; less primary angioplasty; less aspirin treatment; less beta blocker treatment; less heparin treatment; and less bypass graft surgery.

13. How does CAD differ in women?

Coronary artery disease is the #1 killer among women. In fact, six times as many women die of coronary artery disease than from breast cancer. Women's estrogenic coronary protection fades soon after menopause. When compared to men, women experience myocardial infarction at a later age. About 56% of women with myocardial infarction are of age 70 or older. Women have more atypical presentations for an acute myocardial infarction than men. Shortness of breath, epigastric discomfort, nausea, vomiting, diaphoresis, and fatigue are not uncommon amongst women in their presentation of acute myocardial infarction. Moreover, women present their symptoms to the physician or to the emergency room much later than men.

The use of aspirin, heparin, and beta blockers are less frequent among women. Thrombolysis when used in women is on an average 14 minutes later.   Unfortunately, women also experience a greater incidence of bleeding complications from thrombolytic agents. Cardiac catheterizations, angioplasty and bypass graft surgery are used less frequently among women. Women have a higher mortality rate than men, and a greater incidence of cardiac rupture and sudden death from thrombolytic therapy.

The medical community is frequently blamed for under-diagnosing and under-treating women with heart disease. We often wonder whether indeed there is a physician bias.

Symptom of chest pain or shortness of breath: The prevalence of CAD is less in women than in men. For example, a 60-year-old man and a 60-year-old woman presenting with identical symptoms of angina, the man has a greater than 90% chance of having significant CAD, whereas the woman has just less than 50%. In general, ER physicians and the community, as a whole, is attuned to the fact of men presenting with AMI or sudden death as their first manifestation of CAD, whereas in women the mode of presentation is atypical.

> There is a certain level of genuine confusion, and a clinically apparent built-in bias among physicians in responding with the same level of urgency in women in comparison to men.

The problem is further complicated by the fact that initial screening tests, like stress tests, have reduced sensitivity in women, making diagnosis more difficult. Even with more advanced diagnostic tests like stress echocardiography and dobutamine echocardiography, it is impossible to reach a high level of diagnostic accuracy in women. There are more false-positive and false-negative results in women, leading to errors on either side of the spectrum. That is one of the reasons why women get less coronary angiograms than men. When they do get an angiogram for similar indications, women have more percentages of normal coronary arteries than men.

Non-invasive diagnostic tests for CAD in women

Test	Sensitivity	Specificity
Exercise Test	25% (very poor)	80%
Dobutamine stress test	40%(poor)	81%
Stress Echocardiogram	65-70% (average)	80%

Hence, there is a certain level of genuine confusion, and a clinically apparent built-in bias among physicians in responding with the same level of urgency in women in comparison to men. However, it has been proven beyond doubt that women in general are about 40% less likely to be referred for an angiogram no matter what. In particular, African-American females are about 60% less frequently referred for coronary angiograms than Caucasian males, suggesting a clear signal of physician bias. This is an area where the medical profession has to pay a lot more attention in giving credit to atypical presentations of CAD, choosing the right diagnostic test, and showing greater willingness to refer women for angiograms.

> African-American females are about 60% less frequently referred for coronary angiograms than Caucasian males, suggesting a clear signal of physician bias.

When it comes to hypertension are women different?

For hemoglobin, hematocrit, body surface area, and several other physiological and biochemical values, the female has a separate norm. It is my impression that "normal blood pressure" in a woman is about 5-10 mm lower than a man. Therefore, it is my personal belief that when we set standards for hypertension, the upper limit must be 130/85 for a woman rather than 140/90. Systolic blood pressure of 130-139 and diastolic blood pressure of 85-89 must be considered as high-normal. However, women with high-normal blood pressure are noted to have three times more myocardial infarctions and two times more strokes than normotensive females. Therefore, these high-normal blood pressures must be identified as such, and treated by diet, salt restriction, exercise, and pharmacological agents if needed.

14. <u>Can coronary artery disease (CAD) be cured?</u>

Unfortunately, CAD is a permanent as well as progressive disease of the coronary system. The process of atherosclerosis (cholesterol build-up in the vessels producing premature aging) is somewhat universal in a given individual with affliction in the coronary, cerebral, renal, and peripheral arterial systems.

If the patient has very high cholesterol, aggressive treatment with cholesterol lowering agents has clearly shown quite significant reduction in the incidence of myocardial infarction (up to 34% reduction of MI). The overall mortality rate is also reduced by 30%. In addition, a 37% reduction is noted in revascularization procedures such as open-heart surgery and PTCA. The famous Simvastatin Survival Study (4S Study-Merck 1994), which showed the aforementioned beneficial effects with cholesterol reduction have revolutionized the treatment of patients with hypercholesterolemia. Similar beneficial effects have also been observed with Pravachol (Bristol-Myers Squibb). In some patients with documented coronary atherosclerosis and hypercholesterolemia, aggressive reduction of cholesterol has shown some resolution in the atherosclerotic process, and reduction in the degree of coronary stenosis. However, the short-term effect of these medications is to passivate the cholesterol plaque with its anti-inflammatory properties, thereby reducing the chance of erosion and rupture.

Thus, the natural history of CAD can be modified. In some instances, the degree of the lesion can be reversed, and the complications can be reduced. However, atherosclerosis is considered to be a permanent affliction once it has occurred.

15. <u>What about chelation therapy?</u>

I had a couple of patients coming to me with stories of miraculous cure of coronary artery disease following chelation therapy. However, further inquiry into the case history did not show any strong clinical or angiographic evidence of coronary artery disease before the chelation therapy, or resolution of the blockages after the chelation therapy.

Miracles are events of the past that lack predictability, accountability, or reproducibility.

It is my feeling that some kind of a miracle can be used in the management of coronary artery disease in several cases; however, such a miracle is yet to come.

Chapter Eight

Cardiac External Counterpulsation

(CECP)

I believe that EECP* has great potential, and could be particularly applicable to patients who are not candidates for revascularization, but who continue to have repetitive episodes of myocardial ischemia.

Richard Conti, M.D.
Cardiology Professor of Medicine
Journal of American College of Cardiology, vol. 33, #7, 1999.

*Enhanced External Counterpulsation

Coronary artery disease with angina or angina equivalent symptoms is usually treated with antianginal medications (aspirin, nitrates, beta blockers, calcium channel blocking agents, etc.), coronary angioplasty, stenting, or coronary artery bypass surgery. But there still remains a very large pool of patients where all these options have run out, yet they continue to have disabling angina.

In our pursuit for alternative options to treat these patients, several other modalities of treatment have evolved such as transmyocardial laser revascularization, transcutaneous electrical nerve stimulation, spinal cord stimulation, and CECP.

CECP, the subject in point here, is meant for the following subset of patients:

a. Patients who have had multiple angioplasties and coronary artery bypass surgeries, and that such procedures are no longer feasible.
b. Contraindication for bypass graft surgery due to other medical conditions.
c. Coronary anatomy is unsuitable for additional PTCA, stenting, or CABG (diffuse vasculopathy).
d. Severe microvascular coronary artery disease where PTCA or CABG is not an option.
e. When all arterial and venous conduits have been used, and additional bypass surgery is not possible.
f. Patients who are just fed up with multiple procedures with no longstanding benefit.
g. Patients who do not want PTCA or CABG by choice.

What is CECP?

CECP is a novel non-pharmacological outpatient treatment for angina secondary to coronary artery disease. It is a fairly complex cardiac-assist device that will increase the coronary blood flow by increasing the diastolic pressure in the central aorta over and above the systolic pressure by synchronized squeezing of the lower extremity vessels in the diastolic phase of the cardiac cycle.

In order to understand CECP, you should know the fundamentals of coronary circulation. Coronary arteries are the first pair of arteries originating from the root of the aorta that supply the whole cardiac musculature. All the organs of the body (brain, lungs, kidneys, etc.), except the heart muscle, receive most of its blood supply during the contraction phase (cardiac systole) of the left ventricle. The pulse we feel in the arteries is that systolic impulse. However, in systole, the heart muscle is in a contracted state, and therefore blood flow is minimal in the coronary vascular bed (Fig. 20A). In diastole the heart muscle relaxes, and the coronary vascular bed will fill up with all the blood it can with a sucking effect from the aortic root (Fig. 20B). Therefore, if we can selectively increase the diastolic blood pressure at the aortic root, we can increase the coronary filling, thereby the coronary circulation at large.

Since the 1960s, scientists have been working to achieve this goal of increasing the diastolic pressure in the aortic root by an assist device. The result was the perfection of the intra-aortic balloon pump, which is commonly used in situations like cardiogenic shock. However, intra-aortic balloon pump is a highly invasive technique with the introduction of a large tube and balloon system into the central aorta, and its use is limited to the Cardiac Catheterization Labs, Operation Suites, as well as Intensive Care Units.

CECP is an ingenious external cardiac-assist device that came to fruition after 40 years of research and trials. The equipment is totally noninvasive, and is used in an outpatient setting in the cardiologist's office. Patients are very carefully screened and selected for this therapy. During the treatment, the patient lies down on a special bed. Three pairs of rapidly inflatable and deflatable pneumatic cuffs (pressure suits) are applied to the calves, thighs, and girdle. Continuous electrocardiographic monitoring for cardiac rhythm, and direct plethysmographic measurements for blood pressures are now established. During the diastolic phase of the cardiac cycle, the CECP pressure cuffs are rapidly inflated in sequence starting from the calf, the thigh, and finally the buttocks (Figs. 18A, B, C, D and E). The cuffs are inflated with a pressure of 250-300 mmHg. With this squeezing mechanism, blood is forcefully propelled back to the central aorta creating a retrograde blood flow during diastole. This diastolic augmentation of blood pressure, and the resultant increase in blood flow through the coronary arteries, and finally to the myocardium is the crux of this treatment modality. Similarly, the venous system is also squeezed in a similar fashion resulting in increased venous return to the right atrium and right ventricle, eventually improving the cardiac output.

During the systolic phase of the cardiac cycle, the pressure cuffs are rapidly deflated. At this stage, the compressed and under-filled vessels of the lower extremity will quickly dilate and re-conform sucking in blood from the central aorta. This reduction in the afterload of the left ventricle augments emptying of the contents of the left ventricle into the aorta much more effectively, thereby improving the cardiac output. This synchronized inflation and deflation sequence is continued for one hour as the treatment is continued. Normally, the treatment is scheduled one hour per day for 35 days spread over seven weeks.

The hemodynamic effects and the clinical benefits

Several studies have shown that CECP clearly improves the cardiac function from many different standpoints as briefly mentioned here. First of all, direct plethysmographic studies show that the diastolic augmentation is quite remarkable and comparable to intra-aortic balloon pump treatment. This increase in diastolic pressure at the aortic root certainly augments the pressure as well as the velocity of flow through the coronary arteries. This enhanced diastolic perfusion pressure and velocity facilitates the opening of new collaterals, and in my opinion transforms recruitable dormant collaterals into functional collaterals. The formation of these new collaterals will activate a very large number of endothelial cells, which will in turn liberate nitric oxide and prostacyclin, two important hormones responsible for vasodilatation at the microvasculature level of the coronary arterial system. Although CECP does not affect the ejection fraction or systolic indices in any significant way, a very modest increase in cardiac output, particularly the forward stroke volume by up to 12% has been noted in some selected studies. We have seen a reduction in pulmonary capillary wedge pressure as the treatment has progressed in patients.

Certainly, the coronary circulation increases in diastole by 20-40%. In addition, the carotid, renal, as well as hepatic flow volume have been increased by 20-25%.

Patients who have completed a 35-day treatment have noted increased exercise tolerance with increased exercise duration, as well as increased time to ischemia (1.0 mm of ST depression) for a routine treadmill test. In addition, we also have noted better myocardial oxygen utilization (rate pressure product) at peak exercise, as well as better rate pressure product at 1.0 mm ST depression with exercise. Radionuclide scintigraphic studies have demonstrated reversible myocardial ischemia in several studies. It also has clearly shown increased perfusion of the myocardium following a treatment course. However, no change has been noted on fixed perfusion abnormalities. In all of these cases, it is most important that at least one artery be open to gain the benefits from CECP treatment.

From the clinical standpoint, patients have experienced less anginal episodes, less requirement for Nitroglycerin, increased exercise duration, and better exercise duration to develop 1.0 mm ST depression on exercise treadmill test.

Long-term effects

The mechanism of long-term beneficial effect is unclear. However, there is a reasonable body of evidence that suggests the beneficial effect from one set of treatment continues as long as five years. Formation of new collaterals and recruitment of dormant collaterals into functional circulation are speculated. We have also noted a preservation of this benefit on a long-term basis from thallium scintigraphic studies.

Adverse effects

CECP produces a fair amount of minor adverse effects. No mortality has been reported so far. Some patients do not tolerate the look, noise, as well as the complexity of the machine, and therefore withdraw from the treatment. Skin aberrations, bruises, leg pain, paresthesia, anxiety, dizziness, tinnitus, headache, GI symptoms, palpitations, and angina have been reported. In general, about 5% of the patients enrolled for the treatment discontinue it due to these side effects.

Patients who are not candidates for CECP treatment

Not all patients are ideal candidates for CECP treatment, although the indications are slowly evolving as we gain more experience with this treatment modality. As it stands now, severe congestive cardiac failure, chronic atrial fibrillation, myocardial infarction within the last three months, recurrent DVT, varicose veins, stasis ulcers, severe peripheral vascular disease, aortic insufficiency, uncontrolled hypertension of more than 180/100 mmHg, long-term anticoagulation, or bleeding diathesis are considered to be contraindications. All patients who undergo this treatment must have a coronary angiogram. Non-bypassed left main coronary artery disease with more than 50% stenosis is also considered to be a contraindication.

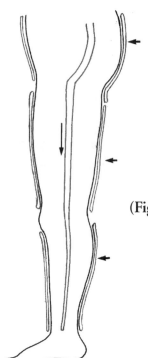

Schematics of the arterial circulation to the lower limbs. At the
end of cardiac systole, the arteries are
fully filled and carry blood down-
stream to the tissues. The long arrow
shows direction of blood flow. The
small arrow shows deflated pressure
cuffs.

(Fig. 18A)

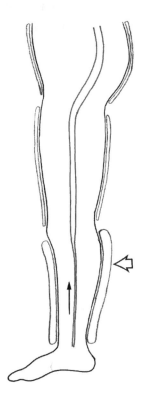

(Fig. 18B)

The early diastolic phase of the
cardiac cycle. The cuffs against the
calf muscles are inflated as shown by
the large arrow. The small arrow
shows compression of the arteries in
the calf, and reversal of blood flow
towards the heart.

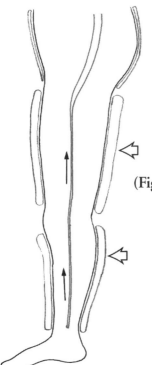

Mid diastolic phase of the cardiac cycle. The large arrow shows the inflated cuffs of the calf and thigh. The small arrow shows compression of the arteries in the calf and thigh with reversal of blood flow towards the heart.

(Fig. 18C)

(Fig. 18D)

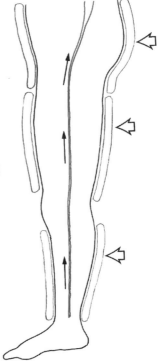

The late diastolic phase of the cardiac cycle. The cuffs against the calves, thighs, and buttocks are now inflated, as shown by the large arrows. The resultant arterial compression and the reversal of blood flow towards the heart are shown by the long arrows.

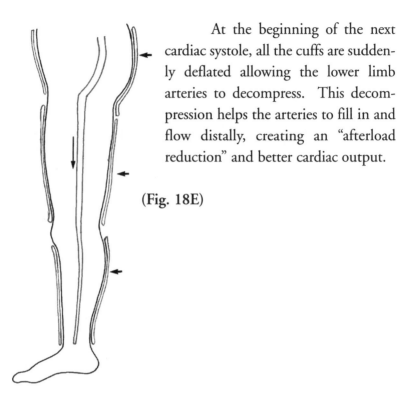

At the beginning of the next cardiac systole, all the cuffs are suddenly deflated allowing the lower limb arteries to decompress. This decompression helps the arteries to fill in and flow distally, creating an "afterload reduction" and better cardiac output.

(Fig. 18E)

This sequential inflation of the cuffs in the legs and buttocks produces a reversal of blood flow towards the central aorta producing the diastolic augmentation of the central aortic pressure.

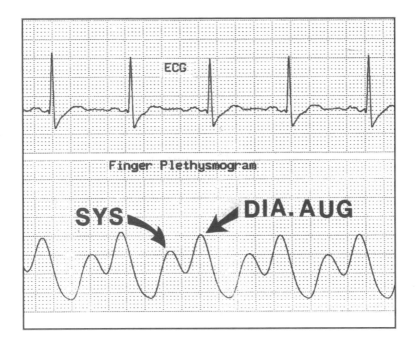

(**Fig. 19**) Simultaneous electrocardiogram and finger plethysmogram from a 68-year-old patient recorded during CECP treatment. Systolic pressure 124 mmHg.   Peak diastolic augmented blood pressure 160 mmHg.   This diastolic augmentation is achieved by the sequential inflation of the lower limb and buttock cuffs during diastolic phase of the cardiac cycle.   This diastolic augmentation certainly increases coronary flow velocity, which is the goal of this treatment.

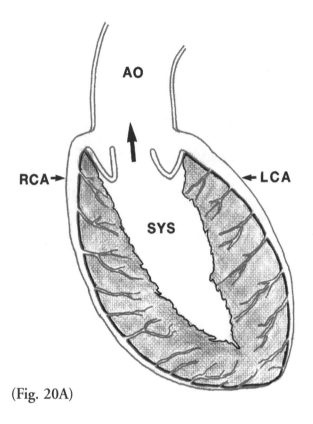

(Fig. 20A)

Schematics of coronary circulation during cardiac systole of the left ventricle.

In systole, the heart muscle contracts, the aortic valve opens, and about 60-70% of its contained blood is ejected into the aorta. The small arteries that supply the heart muscle are squeezed in that contractile process, thereby markedly reducing the coronary blood flow in cardiac systole.

AO-aorta. *RCA*-right coronary artery. *LCA*-left circumflex artery.

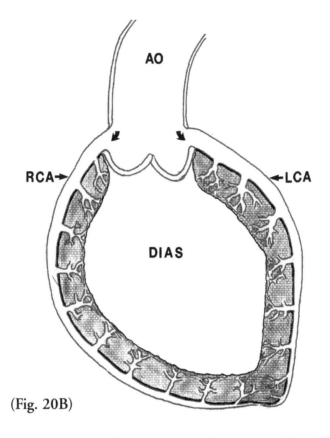

(Fig. 20B)

Schematics of coronary circulation in cardiac diastole (the filling phase of the left ventricle). The aortic valve is now closed. The mitral valve (not shown in the schematics) opens into the left ventricle. The cardiac muscle relaxes. The intramyocardial pressure is now relieved. The small coronary vessels dilated creating a relatively negative intramyocardial pressure. The combination of these factors helps the coronary arteries to "suck up" more blood from the aortic root, markedly boosting the coronary blood flow in diastole. In fact, the coronary blood flow in diastole improves by 400-500% when compared to systole.

Glossary

ACE   Angiotensin-converting enzyme. An enzyme that regulates your blood pressure. ACE is elevated in heart failure.

ACEI Angiotensin-converting enzyme inhibitor. A group of medications used to treat hypertension and heart failure.

ACLS Advanced Cardiac Life Support.

AMI   Acute myocardial infarction.
Heart attack – Heart seizure.

Angina Chest pain originating from the heart due to spasm or occlusion of the coronary arteries.

Angioplasty   The procedure by which a clogged vessel (e.g., coronary artery) is opened up with a balloon catheter.

BCLS Basic Cardiac Life Support.

CABG Coronary artery bypass graft surgery. See Chapter Seven, Question 8, Page 140.

CAD   Coronary artery disease. Synonymous to buildup of cholesterol in the coronary arteries.

Cardioversion The application of electrical discharge directly to the chest wall, to convert an abnormal chaotic rhythm of the heart to a normal rhythm.

CAT Computerized Axial Tomography. A special X-ray that will show details of the human body, head, chest, etc.

CECP Cardiac External CounterPulsation.

COPD Chronic Obstructive Pulmonary Disease.

CPR Cardiopulmonary resuscitation.

CVD Cardiovascular diseases. Comprises coronary artery disease, hypertension and stroke.

Defibrillation Is synonymous with cardioversion.

Defibrillator Refer to Chapter Six, Section 2, Page 93.

ECG (EKG) Electrocardiogram.

EECP Synonymous with CECP.

ETT Exercise treadmill test.

FHH Familial Homozygous Hypercholesterolemia.

HDL High-density lipoprotein.
　　　　Good cholesterol.

HRV   Heart rate variability. Refer to Chapter Seven, Question 12, Page 159.

Hypertension Sustained elevation of blood pressure above the normal range. Refer to Chapter Three, Section 1, Page 34.

ICU   Intensive Care Unit.

LAD   Left anterior descending artery.

LCX   Left circumflex artery.

LDL   Low-density lipoprotein.
           Bad cholesterol.

LIMA Left internal mammary artery.

LM   Left main.

OB/GYN   Obstetrics and Gynecology.

PTCA Percutaneous transluminal coronary angioplasty.

PTCI Synonymous with PTCA.

RCA   Right coronary artery.

RIMA Right internal mammary artery.

SCA   Sudden cardiac arrest.

SCD   Sudden cardiac death.

SCDS Sudden cardiac death syndrome.

SVG   Saphenous vein graft.

V. Fib Ventricular fibrillation.

VT   Ventricular tachycardia.